Multicultural Therapy

Theories of Psychotherapy Series

Theories of Psychotherapy Series

Matt Englar-Carlson, Series Editor

Multicultural Therapy

A Practice Imperative

Melba J. T. Vasquez and
Josephine D. Johnson

 AMERICAN PSYCHOLOGICAL ASSOCIATION

Published by
American Psychological Association
750 First Street, NE
Washington, DC 20002
https://www.apa.org

Order Department
https://www.apa.org/pubs/books
order@apa.org

In the U.K., Europe, Africa, and the Middle East, copies may be ordered from Eurospan
https://www.eurospanbookstore.com/apa
info@eurospangroup.com

Typeset in Minion by Circle Graphics, Inc., Reisterstown, MD

Printer: Gasch Printing, Odenton, MD
Cover Designer: Beth Schlenoff Design, Bethesda, MD
Cover Art: *Lily Rising*, 2005, oil and mixed media on panel in craquelure frame, by Betsy Bauer

Library of Congress Cataloging-in-Publication Data

Names: Vasquez, Melba Jean Trinidad, author. | Johnson, Josephine D., author.
Title: Multicultural therapy : a practice imperative / by Melba J. T. Vasquez and Josephine D. Johnson.
Description: Washington, DC : American Psychological Association, [2022] | Series: Theories of psychotherapy | Includes bibliographical references and index.
Identifiers: LCCN 2021047277 (print) | LCCN 2021047278 (ebook) | ISBN 9781433836480 (paperback) | ISBN 9781433839313 (ebook)
Subjects: LCSH: Cultural psychiatry. | Psychotherapy—Cross-cultural studies. | BISAC: PSYCHOLOGY / Psychotherapy / General | PSYCHOLOGY / Ethnopsychology
Classification: LCC RC455.4.E8 V37 2022 (print) | LCC RC455.4.E8 (ebook) | DDC 616.89/14—dc23
LC record available at https://lccn.loc.gov/2021047277
LC ebook record available at https://lccn.loc.gov/2021047278

https://doi.org/10.1037/0000279-000

Printed in the United States of America

10 9 8 7 6 5 4 3 2 1

To my parents, Joe and Ofelia Vasquez,
who taught us to value culture, family, and education;
and my spouse, Jim Miller, the best ally in the world!
—*MJTV*

To my remarkable husband, Wayne;
and my phenomenal daughters, Lindsay and Chelsea.
—*JDJ*

Contents

Series Preface

Matt Englar-Carlson

Some might argue that in the contemporary clinical practice of psychotherapy, the focus on evidence-based intervention and effective outcome has overshadowed theory in importance. Maybe. But at the same time, it is clear that psychotherapists adopt and practice according to one theory or another because their experience, and decades of empirical evidence, suggests that having a sound theory of psychotherapy leads to greater therapeutic success. Theory is fundamental in guiding psychotherapists in understanding *why* people behave, think, and feel in certain ways, and it provides the guidance to then contemplate *what* a client can do to instigate meaningful change. Still, the role of theory in the helping process itself can be hard to explain. This narrative about solving problems may help convey theory's importance:

> Aesop tells the fable of the sun and wind having a contest to decide who was the most powerful. From above the earth, they spotted a person walking down the street, and the wind said that he bet he could get his coat off. The sun agreed to the contest. The wind blew, and the person held on tightly to his coat. The more the wind blew, the tighter the person held on to his coat. The sun said it was his turn. He put all of his energy into creating warm sunshine, and soon the person took off his coat.

What does a competition between the sun and the wind to get the person to remove a coat have to do with theories of psychotherapy? This deceptively simple story highlights the importance of theory as the precursor to any effective intervention—and hence to a favorable outcome. Without a guiding theory, a psychotherapist might treat the symptom without understanding the role of the individual. Or we might create power conflicts with our clients and not understand that, at times, indirect means of helping (sunshine) are often as effective as—if not more so than—direct ones (wind). In the absence of theory, a psychotherapist might lose track of the treatment rationale and instead get caught up in, for example, social correctness and not wanting to do something that looks too simple.

What exactly *is* theory? The *APA Dictionary of Psychology, Second Edition* defines theory as "a principle or body of interrelated principles that purports to explain or predict a number of interrelated phenomena" (VandenBos, 2015, p. 1081). In psychotherapy, a theory is a set of principles used to explain human thought and behavior, including what causes people to change. In practice, a theory frames the goals of therapy and specifies how to pursue them. Haley (1997) noted that a theory of psychotherapy ought to be simple enough for the average psychotherapist to understand but comprehensive enough to account for a wide range of eventualities. Furthermore, a theory guides action toward successful outcomes while generating hope in both the psychotherapist and client that recovery is possible.

Theory is the compass that allows psychotherapists to navigate the vast territory of clinical practice. In the same ways that navigational tools have been modified to adapt to advances in thinking and ever-expanding territories to explore, theories of psychotherapy have evolved over time to account for advances in science and technology. The different schools of theories are commonly referred to as *waves*—the first wave of psychodynamic theories (i.e., Adlerian, psychoanalytic), the second wave of learning theories (i.e., behavioral, cognitive-behavioral), the third wave of humanistic theories (i.e., person centered, gestalt, existential), the fourth wave of feminist and multicultural theories, and the fifth wave of postmodern and constructivist theories (i.e., narrative, constructivist). In many ways, these waves represent how psychotherapy has adapted and responded to changes in psychology, society, and epistemology, as well as to changes in the nature of psychotherapy itself. The wide variety of theories is also a testament to the different ways in which the same human behavior can be conceptualized depending on the view one espouses (Frew & Spiegler, 2012). Our theories of psychotherapy are also challenged to expand beyond the primarily Western worldview endemic in most psychotherapy theories and the practice of psychotherapy itself. That revision and correction requires theories and psychotherapists to become more inclusive of the full range of human diversity to reflect an understanding of human behavior that accounts for a client's context, identity, and intersectionality (American Psychological Association, 2017). To that end, psychotherapy and the theories that guide it are dynamic and responsive to the changing world around us.

With these two concepts in mind—the central importance of theory and the natural evolution of theoretical thinking—the APA Theories of Psychotherapy Series was developed. This series was created by my father (Jon Carlson) and me. Although educated in different eras, we both had a love of theory and often spent time discussing the range of complex ideas that drove each model. Even though my father identified strongly as an Adlerian and I was parented and raised from the Adlerian perspective, my father always espoused an appreciation for other theories and theorists—and that is something I picked up from him. As university faculty members teaching courses on the theories of psychotherapy, we wanted to create learning materials that not only highlighted the essence of the major theories for professionals and professionals in training but also clearly brought the reader up-to-date on the current status of the models, future directions with an emphasis on the inclusive application of the theories with clients representing the range of identities. Often in books on theory, the biography of the original theorist overshadows the evolution of the model. In contrast, our intent was to highlight the contemporary uses of the theories as well as their history and context—both past and present.

As this project began, we faced two immediate decisions: which theories to address and who best to present them. We assessed graduate-level theories of psychotherapy courses to see which theories are being taught, and we explored popular scholarly books, articles, and conferences to determine which theories draw the most interest. We then developed a dream list of authors from among the best minds in contemporary theoretical practice. To that end, each author in the series is one of the leading proponents of that approach as well as a knowledgeable practitioner. We asked each author to review the core constructs of the theory, bring the theory into the modern sphere of clinical practice by looking at it through a context of evidence-based practice, and clearly illustrate how the theory looks in application.

This is the 25th title in the series, and many titles are now in their second edition. Each title can stand alone or can be put together with a few other titles to create materials for a course in psychotherapy theories. This option allows instructors to create a course featuring the approaches they believe are the most salient today. To support this end, APA Books has also developed videos for each of the approaches to demonstrate the theory in practice with a real client. Many of the videos show psychotherapy over six sessions with the same client. Contact APA Books for a complete list of available video programs (https://www.apa.org/pubs/videos).

Of all the titles in this series, *Multicultural Therapy* is possibly the most timely and critical monograph. It is difficult for me to conceptualize the influence of the critique that multiculturally focused scholars had and continue to have on the theory, science, and practice of psychotherapy itself. Beyond simply being the fourth wave of theories of psychotherapy, multicultural therapy and the ethical imperatives to provide equitably and socially just clinical practice shape all the preceding and subsequent theories of psychotherapy.

Communicating the vast range of multicultural psychology and counselor scholarship is a monumental task, yet Melba J. T. Vasquez and Josephine D. Johnson are more than up to it. Readers of this book are encouraged to start from a place of cultural humility as student, scholar, and practitioner. Cultural humility requires ongoing self-reflection and self-critique, particularly in identifying patterns of unintentional and intentional racism in the practice of psychotherapy and in the ways that each of us delivers clinical services. In essence, cultural humility adopts a balanced approach to holding on to professional expertise and knowledge while asking questions that challenge one to listen more deeply and to recognize when one's knowledge, beliefs, or practices are inaccurate or require adaptation to meet the full range of cultural identities and histories. Fisher noted that cultural humility adopts a questioning stance of "What if this is not the whole picture?" or "What might I be missing?" (Owen et al., 2015, as cited in Fisher, 2020, p. 60) as a means of opening one up to new ideas or modifying existing beliefs into culturally responsive ones. *Multicultural Therapy* and *The Basics of Psychotherapy* (Wampold, 2019) serve as the entry points for any of the other monographs in this series.

REFERENCES

American Psychological Association. (2017). *Multicultural guidelines: An ecological approach to context, identity, and intersectionality.* http://www.apa.org/about/policy/multicultural-guidelines.pdf

Fisher, E. S. (2020). Cultural humility as a form of social justice: Promising practices for global school psychology training. *School Psychology International, 41*(1), 53–66. https://doi.org/10.1177/0143034319893097

Frew, J., & Spiegler, M. (2012). *Contemporary psychotherapies for a diverse world* (1st rev. ed.). Routledge.

Haley, J. (1997). *Leaving home: The therapy of disturbed young people.* Routledge.

VandenBos, G. (2015). *APA dictionary of psychology* (2nd ed.). American Psychological Association.

Wampold, B. E. (2019). *The basics of psychotherapy: An introduction to theory and practice* (2nd ed.). https://doi.org/10.1037/0000117-000

How to Use This Book With APA Psychotherapy Videos

Each book in the Theories of Psychotherapy Series is usually paired with a video that demonstrates the theory applied in actual therapy with a real client. Many videos feature the author of the book as the guest therapist, allowing students to see an eminent scholar and practitioner putting the theory they write about into action. Because of the range of skills, interventions, and considerations addressed in the *Multicultural Therapy* monograph, multiple videos are recommended.

The video programs have several features that make them excellent tools for learning more about theoretical concepts. Most programs have a brief introductory discussion recapping the basic features of the theory or concept being demonstrated. This allows viewers to review the key aspects of the approach about which they have just read.

Many videos feature volunteer clients in unedited psychotherapy sessions. This provides a unique opportunity to get a sense of the look and feel of real psychotherapy, something that written case examples and transcripts sometimes cannot convey. Other videos feature actors in scripted sessions that clearly illustrate the concept being presented.

The books and videos together make a powerful teaching tool for showing how theoretical principles affect practice. In the case of this book, the video *Multicultural Therapy Over Time*, which features the first author as the guest expert, provides a vivid example of how this approach looks in practice. This program contains six full sessions of psychotherapy over time, giving viewers a chance to see how clients respond to the application of the theory over the course of several sessions.

Other suggested videos include:

- *Cultural Humility in Therapy.* In this video, Dr. Cirleen DeBlaere demonstrates cultural humility working with a client who has experienced tragic loss in her life. In a postsession discussion, Dr. Jesse Owen talks with Dr. DeBlaere about the demonstration and the usefulness of fostering cultural humility in therapy.
- *The Dynamics of Power and Privilege in Psychotherapy.* In this video, Malin Fors demonstrates and discusses clinical topics associated with power and privilege in psychotherapy, such as voluntary and involuntary self-disclosure, similarities between patient and therapist, and internalized oppression, and then highlights specific moments in the demonstration session when client–therapist power dynamics come into play.
- *Reflections on Race and Ethnicity in the Therapeutic Setting.* In this program, four therapists known for their culturally adaptive work discuss ways to honor differences in identity and address the effects of prejudice in psychotherapy. Clinical demonstrations show how to address race nondefensively with clients who have recently experienced an incident of prejudice against them.

For more information, please visit APA Videos (https://www.apa.org/pubs/videos/).

Acknowledgments

Several years ago, I (Melba) was honored to be invited to be the author of the *Multicultural Therapy* monograph in the American Psychological Association (APA) Theories of Psychotherapy Series. I accepted the invitation, but several events, projects, and life experiences "got in the way." I worked on drafts of the monograph off and on, and the importance of this topic weighed heavily on me. It was not until I invited coauthor Jo Johnson to join me that the productivity increased significantly. I have always worked best when in collaboration with others, and Jo has been an inspiring, fun, and joyful cowriter. I am inordinately grateful to Jo for her significant contributions.

We spent a year sharing drafts, chapters, and sections, and we decided to invite our friend and colleague Cynthia de las Fuentes to serve as our editor. We are both so appreciative of the expert editing and numerous suggestions made by Cynthia. She contributed to a positive working process that lightened the load and underscored the value of the project.

We are all grateful for the patience and reviews of series editor Matt Englar-Carlson and regret that Jon Carlson, his father and coeditor, did not live to see our final product. We are also exceedingly appreciative of the gentle nudges, support, and sharp reviews of APA editor Kristen Knight as well as Susan Reynolds, who was our initial APA editor. We also appreciate the work of other APA staff. The feedback from Matt, Kristen, and three anonymous reviewers was helpful in our final revisions of the monograph.

The three of us are grateful for the influences of the many scholars, professors, colleagues, clients, and students who have significantly informed our work. This was a true labor of love. The subject of multicultural psychology and multicultural (psycho)therapy is important and constantly evolving, and we truly hope we have contributed in a beneficial way to the scholarship on this critical topic.

We also want to thank our families and friends who supported our work with this and numerous other projects over the years. Their support allows us to spend time doing the work we value, and we are lucky to have them in our lives!

Multicultural Therapy

1

Introduction

Multicultural psychology is a theoretical framework that underpins *multicultural psychotherapy*, which is the provision of competent and ethical interventions to culturally diverse clients (D. W. Sue et al., 1992). While multicultural competence in psychotherapy has become part of the mainstream fundamental knowledge and skill set required for effective practice for more than 5 decades (Ho & McDowell, 1973; T. B. Smith & Trimble, 2016; D. W. Sue et al., 1992; S. Sue et al., 2009), more than ever, it now requires increased knowledge and sophistication on the part of the professional. Because all behaviors are learned and displayed in particular cultural contexts, multiculturally competent therapists must be prepared to address their own behaviors and cultural assumptions, those of their clients, and the relationship between the two in the contexts of their sociocultural histories and therapeutic relationships. A Glossary of Key Terms is included at the end of the book, after the last chapter, and may be helpful to the reader.

https://doi.org/10.1037/0000279-001
Multicultural Therapy: A Practice Imperative, by M. J. T. Vasquez and J. D. Johnson

UNDERSTANDING MULTICULTURAL THERAPY

Our definition of *multicultural therapy* (for the purposes of this monograph, *multicultural [psycho]therapy* and *multicultural counseling* are used interchangeably, as are *[psycho]therapists* and *counselors*) integrates concepts developed by others (e.g., Fuertes et al., 2015; Pedersen, 2002; Tylor, 1920). Specifically, we believe it is the practice of psychotherapy informed by multicultural philosophies and theories, grounded in multicultural scholarship on the psychology of race and ethnicity, that leads psychotherapists and their clients toward culturally appropriate strategies and solutions that advance transformation and social change in their personal lives and in their relationships with their social, emotional, and political environments (L. S. Brown, 1994).

Importantly, multicultural therapy is based on models that identify the toxic effects of pervasive bias on the psychotherapy process itself, including stereotyping, devaluing, disempowering, pathologizing, doubting or minimizing experiences of marginalization, and/or assuming the incompetence of clients. It includes a commitment to the elimination of implicit biases within ourselves and our clients because we know of those biases' deleterious effects on each other and on the psychotherapeutic relationship (L. S. Brown, 2016). Multicultural therapy, at its best, is inherently strengths based and designed to focus on the resilience of our clients and communities (Asnaani & Hofmann, 2012; P. A. Hays, 2009; Peterson & Seligman, 2004; Snyder et al., 2003).

Using Pedersen's (2002) ethnographic, demographic, status, and affiliation social systems framework, we define *culture* broadly, appreciating Tylor's (1920) foundational definition that includes "knowledge, belief, art, morals, law, custom, and any other capabilities and habits acquired by man as a member of society" (p. 1). We further define *multicultural* as encompassing several cultural and ethnic groups within a society and one's own person as well as the intersectionality of those identities.

This monograph pays particular attention to racial and ethnic identities while additionally exploring the intersectionality of a variety of strands of identity that are also aspects of individuals' experiences, including gender, sexual attraction, social class, and ability. The intersectionality

4

framework asks practitioners as well as researchers to consider categories of identity, difference, and (dis)advantage with a new lens. Although early articulations of intersectionality focused on the experiences of groups holding multiple disadvantaged identities (e.g., Melville, 1980), we acknowledge that everyone occupies multiple categories (e.g., gender, race, class, ability) simultaneously. Consequently, the concept of intersectionality can also inform how privileged identities are understood (Cole, 2009) and which identities (privileged and not) are salient according to the varying contexts of our lives (de las Fuentes, 2012).

The research and theory underlying multicultural therapies have undergone significant growth in the past 5 decades. The Association for Multicultural Counseling and Development, for example, endorsed the Multicultural and Social Justice Counseling Competencies (Ratts et al., 2016), which revised the original Multicultural Counseling Competencies developed by D. W. Sue et al. (1992). The revision highlighted the intersection of identities and the dynamics of power, privilege, and oppression that influence the counseling relationship.

The second and most recent version of *Multicultural Guidelines: An Ecological Approach to Context, Identity, and Intersectionality* (hereinafter, *Multicultural Guidelines*) published by the American Psychological Association (APA; 2017b) was conceptualized to view diversity with intersectionality as their primary scope. In the guidelines, psychotherapists are encouraged to consider individual historical and contextual precursors of identities and how those can be employed to generate more effective methods of intervention (APA, 2017b). Recently adopted professional guidelines address this need. For example, the first guidelines to focus specifically on race and ethnicity since APA's 2003 "Guidelines on Multicultural Education, Training, Research, Practice, and Organizational Change for Psychologists" were overwhelmingly approved in August 2019 by the APA Council of Representatives (i.e., *APA Guidelines on Race and Ethnicity in Psychology*; APA, 2019b), as were the *APA Guidelines for Psychological Practice for People With Low-Income and Economic Marginalization* (APA, 2019a), the first guidelines by the APA to address the needs of low-income people.

Understanding the cultural contexts of behavior is essential to effective and ethical interventions in all areas of psychotherapeutic practice because culture influences the experiences and emotional and behavioral expression of distress, dysfunction, strength, and resilience (American Psychiatric Association, 2013; APA, 2017b; Mosher et al., 2017; T. B. Smith & Trimble, 2016). While the scientific literature is rife with talk about particular groups being disadvantaged in society, it is important to note that various aspects of our identities that contribute to group identities (e.g., gender, race) also reflect strength and resilience.

There are many reasons why multicultural competency, and diversity training in general, should be incorporated into the fabric of mental health training programs and continuing education, rather than as stand-alone courses. Multicultural competence requires appropriate awareness, knowledge, and skills about the intersectionality of the many strands of identity, including not only race and ethnicity but also age, generation, culture, language, gender, ability status, sexual orientation, gender identity, socioeconomic status, religion, spirituality, immigration and citizenship status, education, and employment as well as other variables. Understanding how our own various strands of identity combine to influence our worldviews and experiences, including our work as therapists, is as important as understanding how those of our clients influence their own perceptions. Our strands of identity influence our perceptions of problems and issues, as well as what we consider to be healthy and unhealthy processes and functional and dysfunctional coping strategies.

Our clients' strands of identity may also influence which therapeutic approaches might be most effective for them. An intersectional model of understanding various aspects of identity helps the therapist, and thus clients, understand what aspects of identity are relevant and when those aspects of their lives are salient to the narratives being discussed in therapy. No one person is just one of their identities, just as no one is solely male or female, European American or Asian American, or rich or poor. Therapists must ask themselves: "Which aspects of the client's identities are at the forefront of the presenting problem? Which are background? Which will the client benefit from bringing to the forefront? Which are integrated, fused, or inseparable, and from which does a client deidentify?

How do others react to those aspects of their identities?" Importantly, the therapist must determine which aspects of their own identities are salient and can be used in service of the therapeutic relationship. Furthermore, a therapist must acknowledge when a "mismatch" between their own theoretical orientation, cultural perspectives, and identities is not helpful to clients. Although this monograph focuses on culture, race, and ethnicity, we must also acknowledge other intersecting identities.

There is no rule in place regarding the use of the terms *client* or *patient*. The term *patient* is generally considered to be based on the medical model of mental health and has sometimes been criticized as putting the provider in the expert role. *Client* is a more mutual and humanistic description of the relationship between the provider and person seeking services (Vasquez & Heppner, 2017). The terms in this monograph are used interchangeably or as used by the authors cited.

Since there are multiple definitions of *race* and *ethnicity*, it behooves us to describe our understanding of these terms and their usage in this monograph. Historically, the term *race* was an ascribed category, defining a group of persons with shared genetic, biological, and physical features (Gonzalez et al., 2011; Helms et al., 2005). According to that definition, peoples of African, European, Native or Indigenous, and Asian descents represented different races. However, contemporary usage of the term *race* is more congruent with socially constructed realities rather than those that are biologically determined. Today, we appreciate that the meaning of racial group categories has changed across time and context and that the variability within racial groups far exceeds that between racial groups (Helms et al., 2005).

Ethnicity is a category that reflects a group's common history, including national origin, geography, language, and culture; we must also acknowledge significant variability within groups identified as ethnic groups. For example, those with Latinx/Hispanic ethnicity have common origins in Latin America (Mexico, Central and South America, and various Caribbean islands) but may also have European, Asian, and African origins as well as Indigenous Native American origins (*mestizos*). The terms *race* and *ethnicity* are therefore distinct but not mutually exclusive.

More recently, the term *Black, Indigenous, People of Color* (BIPOC) has emerged in our cultural and professional nomenclature, fueled especially by the Black Lives Matter movement. Although the term *POC* has been widely used as an umbrella term for all people of color, emphasizing Black and Indigenous groups is a contemporary attempt to recognize that, as groups, Black and Indigenous peoples are disproportionately affected by systemic and racial injustices (Clarke, 2020). The BIPOC Project describes its mission to build authentic and lasting solidarity among the groups with a unique relationship to Whiteness. Recognizing that each community is differently shaped and situated depending on intersectional issues and identities, the goal of the BIPOC Project is to undo Native invisibility and anti-Blackness while honoring their legacies and uplifting their humanity. Part of its mission is to dismantle White supremacy and advance racial justice for all communities included in the term (BIPOC Project, 2020). We use various terms to describe people's identities throughout this monograph, but when citing literature, we will use terms used by those authors.

DEVELOPMENT OF MULTICULTURAL COMPETENCE: AWARENESS, KNOWLEDGE, AND SKILLS

Pedersen (2002) described how multicultural competence could be considered in a three-level developmental sequence that can span one's professional life cycle. This sequence includes the development of awareness, knowledge, and skills that is complex, nuanced, and builds upon layers of competency.

Our *awareness* and appreciation of human cultural diversity lead to enhanced attitudes and beliefs of cultural sensitivity and an appreciation of diversity. Ethnocentricity, on the other hand, sees differences as bad, negative, and inferior to one's own cultural and ethnic diversity and can result in pathologizing individuals and groups not perceived to be like theirs. People who hold ethnocentric beliefs frequently engage in insidious biasing and microaggressive behaviors.

White/European American psychotherapists must ask themselves, "What work do I need to do to increase my competence and proficiency in my work with African American/Black, Latinx American/Hispanic, Asian American/Asian, Native American/American Indian, Middle Eastern, North African American (MENA)/Arab, Native Hawaiian or Pacific Islander, immigrants or international individuals and their families?" What about other aspects of identity? These clients may be heterosexual, lesbian, gay, bisexual, gender nonconforming/fluid, and/or transgender, as well as possessing various other strands of identity. Specifically, a question psychotherapists need to explore is, "What are the intersectional concerns of some of these identities on my clients, their families and communities, and their presenting problems?" These are questions that therapists of color must also ask of themselves about their ability to work effectively with clients who are both similar and different from themselves. How do any of us learn to work effectively with people who are different from ourselves in many ways? What aspects of humanity are universal and applicable for each client, and which aspects are unique to the complex, evolving, and highly contextual aspects of race, ethnicity, culture, and other elements of identity?

As alluded to previously, clinicians must be aware of their own identities, in addition to the cultural values assumed within traditional psychology and their theories of wellness, disorder, and interventions, because a lack of awareness of themselves and the underlying values of the tools they use may cause harm to the people they are intending to help (Patterson, 1989; D. W. Sue & Sue, 2008). Therapists, therefore, must continuously increase their understanding and awareness of their own sociocultural identities. For example, we should ask ourselves, "What is the impact of my (non)religious beliefs on my clients? How do my clients perceive my socioeconomic status, and what beliefs do I have about theirs? What values and biases that I hold in my identities affect and influence my work? What are the assumptions of wellness and illness in the theories I use? Are certain identities privileged (e.g., male, heterosexual, cisgender, White, educated, middle class, able bodied) in the theories I use? Can I ethically use them in my work with people of color?"

Cultural knowledge involves the factual understanding of basic anthropological knowledge about cultural variation. For purposes of this context, *culture* refers to the variations associated with race, ethnicity, and/or nationality (Mio et al., 2006; Vontress, 2008). Cultural knowledge can be learned through educational experiences, consultation with cultural experts, and/or meaningful interactions with individuals of diverse backgrounds. The challenge in obtaining knowledge about a particular group is the risk of stereotyping. Women do not all experience their gender in the same way; a Latinx individual does not experience or present her cultural identity as another may, even if they grew up in the same community. Cultural knowledge can be used to assess the degree of application of various cultural values, behaviors, and expectations related to the strands of group identity for each individual. The relevant information about a specific individual can be arrived at through careful, sensitive, and knowledgeable questioning and exploration.

For example, is the Latinx client who takes time off from work to care for her dying mother, who was abusive and neglectful of her throughout her childhood, pathologically codependent and self-abnegating?[1] Or is she strong and resilient in her commitment to her cultural value of honoring her elders? Has the choice resulted in lowering her self-esteem or empowering her with resilience? Does the fact that she is a first-generation immigrant versus fourth generation enter into the equation? These are important issues to explore, and a multiculturally competent therapist knows they are not mutually exclusive but nuanced and temporally situated.

Pope et al. (2021) suggested that understanding culture at a deep, structural level is both important and ethically responsible. They presented a model that describes examples of surface-level culture including food, holidays, celebrations, clothing, visual and performing arts, sports, dancing, language, and the like. They borrowed from Ani (1994) to describe five domains of culture at the deeper levels including ontology (e.g., how reality is defined and who gets to define it), axiology (e.g., which

---

[1] The case examples used throughout this book are fictitious or represent composites of actual cases; the confidentiality of real clients has been maintained.

values are salient and which are nonnegotiable), cosmology (e.g., beliefs about the universe's creation, whether there is a higher power), epistemology (e.g., beliefs about how knowledge is created), and praxis (e.g., how relationships are built with others). Pope et al. suggested that the model can be used with clients to explicitly introduce and explore culture in therapy. Psychotherapists can compare their own responses with those of their clients and determine where their cultures overlap and diverge to help inform the therapeutic process.

Knowledge about the impact of societal racism and discrimination on each individual who shares identities with members of groups oppressed in society is critical in assessing a client's experiences. Racism is foundational in American society and its history. And as a system of power, it continues to structure opportunity, deny privilege, and assign value based on categories of identities. This social interpretation based on how we look leads people to assume what we believe, how we behave, what our potential is, and even what our prognosis is. Racism, sexism, homophobia, and all of the other "-isms" unfairly disadvantage some while unfairly advantaging others (C. P. Jones, 2015). There is a popular quote attributed to Leila Janah, CEO of Sama Group, which describes these disparities well: "Talent is equally distributed, opportunity is not" (retrieved from https://www.azquotes.com/quote/865885). While this may be argued on both counts, there is no doubt that there are clear privileges to being male, White, and resource advantaged.

The negative consequences of racism, discrimination, and bias are horrifically devastating and affect multiple levels, from individual, familial, community, as well as institutional. C. P. Jones (2015) and McGhee (2021) opined how these processes sap the strength of a whole society through the waste of human resources. For example, the wholesale warehousing via imprisonment of Black and Brown men, who could be contributing to their families, communities, and society, has been devastating to communities of color. And years of housing discrimination (e.g., redlining) have contributed to limiting African American, Latinx American, and other diverse groups' ability to own property and create intergenerational wealth when compared with their White American peers.

The individual consequences of racism are also devastating. While a strong sense of self-worth and self-respect are important elements of healthy identity and humanness (Pope & Vasquez, 2016), and various groups are able to provide messages and experiences that buffer some of the negative effects and contribute to resilience (e.g., CNN, 2016), the burden of discrimination is a heavy one. Dignity is as essential to human life as is water, food, and oxygen, and the ability to retain dignity in the face of oppressive hardship is an amazing form of resilience (Hillenbrand, 2010). Yet, to be deprived of one's positive aspects of identity is to be dehumanized and cast below one's value as a person.

The history of slavery in America, stealing the lands of Mexicans in the Southwest, Native American reservation containment, Japanese internments, and Hitler's death camps are examples of racism and oppression of peoples who have subsequently suffered for generations from those experiences. Racism in the United States is not all history, as contemporary political rhetoric, epitomized by inflaming a social climate of hate speech (e.g., Donald Trump's "They're bringing drugs. They're bringing crime. They're rapists"; Gamboa, 2015), threats to minority communities (e.g., Ted Cruz's "We need to empower law enforcement to patrol Muslim neighborhoods before they become radicalized"; Seipel & Sanders, 2016), and Executive Order travel bans for people of certain faiths and races (e.g., Executive Order No. 13769, 82 FR 8977, 2017) provide part of the climate for hate crimes against people of color in the United States. Online forums such as YouTube, Facebook, and Twitter have contributed to "a sudden and rapidly increasing wave of bigotry-spewing videos, hate-oriented affinity groups, racist online commentary, and images encouraging violence against the helpless and minorities—blacks, Asians, Latinos, gays, women, Muslims, Jews—across the Internet and around the world" (Foxman & Wolf, 2013, p. 31). While the specific examples given here may be time bound, hate speech and harmful rhetoric are represented at various times in society. Attention and recognition of how and whether they affect us and our clients will always be important to know.

The COVID-19 pandemic that affected the world beginning in 2020 resulted in an increase in school bullying and verbal and physical violence against individuals perceived to be of Asian descent. Boycotts of Chinese- and Asian-owned restaurants and other businesses have had a chilling impact on personal and communal economies (Asian American Psychological Association [AAPA], 2020). Further, mislabeling of the COVID-19 virus by describing it in geographic or culturally demeaning terms has served to fan the flames of xenophobia and encourage acts of social injustice (AAPA, 2020). These types of sociopolitical realities are important aspects of awareness and knowledge for the multiculturally competent therapist to possess.

People subjected to dehumanizing treatment may experience loneliness, shame, depression, and anxiety (C. P. Jones, 2015) while struggling to maintain optimism and hope. Individuals live with the risks and burdens of being defined by the circumstances of genetics and environments that racists use to belittle and deny equity and justice in a multitude of overt and covert ways. Knowledge of the histories of oppressions, the resulting legacies, and the impact of current oppressive experiences for each individual's cultures and identities is critical for the practitioner who wishes to practice competently.

Skills in multicultural psychotherapy involve cultural competence, the ability to connect emotionally with the patient's cultural perspectives, and the ability to convey culturally appropriate empathy. The culturally competent clinician is also able to provide what Tseng and Streltzer (2004) termed *cultural guidance,* by assessing whether and how a patient's problems are related to cultural variables and experiences and proposing therapeutic approaches based on cultural understandings. Increased insights and understanding, via formal and informal experiences and supervision, about working with those different from us leads to such competence.

For example, domestic violence among Latinx families occurs as frequently as in White European American families, but as with other problems, it is culturally mediated. In one study, Welland and Ribner (2007) developed an intervention with 150 Latinx men who completed a year of court-ordered treatment in Southern California. After listening to how Latinx men thought about manhood (i.e., *machismo*), interpersonal relationships (e.g., *respeto, personalismo*), and family life (e.g., *familismo*), they helped the men in those group therapies identify the aspects of masculinity in Latinx culture that make partner violence unacceptable. Machismo, for example, was reframed as having a sense of responsibility and providing for one's family, not as having misogynistic views according to the Western negative stereotype of Latinx men.

Since clients' sense of therapeutic connection is one of the most significant of the common factors in the success of all psychotherapies (Frank & Frank, 1991; Wampold, 2000), the quality of the alliance between psychotherapist and the client of color is a key area of examination and skill development. The power of the "relationship" in predicting outcome in therapy (Lambert, 2013; Norcross & Lambert, 2011; Walker, 2020) is well established and is even more prominent in multicultural therapy, where modifications to traditional approaches may require a multilayered approach (Fuertes et al., 2015), including additional education or consultation. Potential obstacles to developing a therapeutic alliance, as well as strategies for overcoming them, are important to identify for those wishing to provide competent, ethical services to racial and ethnic minority, international, and immigrant populations. Without question, racial and ethnic diversity among clients pose challenges for all psychotherapists, and these challenges are often subconscious (Greenwald & Banaji, 1995; Vasquez, 2007a, 2007b).

Skills, described above as the ability to connect emotionally with the patient's cultural perspective, may also be viewed from a neuroscience perspective. The view is derived from "working memory," a key theoretical concept in cognitive psychology and neuropsychology. Baddeley's (2000) model of working memory is one of the most influential in the neuroscience field. It is described as having four components: the central executive (attention controller), the phonological loop (holder of speech-based information), a visuospatial sketchpad (holder of visual information), and the episodic buffer—a temporary store that incorporates information from the other components and preserves a sense of time, such that events take place in a continuous sequence. It is simple to align the phonological loop with the importance of attending to a patient's language and expression; to connect the role of the visuospatial sketchpad in keeping track of where a patient is in relation to other objects as they move through the environment, or even to compare the characteristics of the buffer to the therapeutic challenge of focusing on time and the sequence of events in a patient's life and history. These working memory components may have both emic and etic significance, but they are particularly germane to the multicultural therapy imperative to view our patients from multiple facets.

Working memory facilitates comprehension, learning, and reasoning. Essentially, the concept requires the individual to take in and hold information in immediate awareness and then perform a mental operation on that information. Prior to Baddeley (2000), some theorists (Atkinson & Shiffrin, 1968; Broadbent, 1958) had viewed working memory as synonymous with short-term memory, but it is more complex. It has been described simply as holding in mind anything needed to keep in mind (short-term memory) while simultaneously doing something with it. An example might be keeping someone's address in mind while listening to instructions about how to get there.

This concept maps well onto the tripartite multicultural competence sequence of awareness, knowledge, and skills and might be viewed as "cultural working memory." If asked to add two numbers, working memory requires the recall of both numbers before performing the calculation. Cultural working memory requires acquisition of factual knowledge of cultural variation before applying it in individual, meaningful, and fluid ways. The competent therapist must develop awareness of cultural facts in a fundamental way, that is, in the same way that numbers and/or letters must be understood before they can be recalled and manipulated.

The flow of the work of multicultural therapy is of necessity dynamic from both the patient's and the therapist's perspectives. The competent multicultural therapist must have the ability to hold the relevant (and potentially contributing) aspects of their own identities available for processing while at the same time addressing salient features of the patient's identities. There may also be occasions when the task requires the therapist to hold the patient's identities available while processing their own. Perceiving, prioritizing, and processing those vigorous moments in an open and authentic manner requires significant therapeutic skill. It necessitates a commitment to long-term investment in growth and development. It is a reasonable expectation that over time cultural working memory will function much like working memory: quickly and nearly effortlessly.

Being culturally responsive means having a set of defined values and principles and requires individuals and organizations to "have the capacity to value diversity, conduct self-assessment, manage dynamics of difference, institutionalize cultural knowledge, and adapt to diversity and cultural contexts of the communities they serve" (National Center for Cultural Competence, 2004, p. vii). To coin a phrase, therapists must become "ethnoculturally fluent," able to understand and value one culture while honoring and speaking from another. As is further addressed later, responsiveness cannot be assumed because of racial and cultural parity between client and therapist. Sometimes socioeconomic, religious, or political differences are more relevant or challenging.

MULTICULTURAL COMPETENCE AS AN ETHICAL IMPERATIVE

Our professional ethics codes include various imperatives that underlie the importance of competence in psychotherapy with members of various diverse groups (APA, 2017a). At its foundation, multicultural competence requires recognition of the roles of psychotherapists in their work with people who are different from themselves. This awareness is a critical issue in the ethical delivery of psychotherapeutic services. As human beings, we connect more readily to, and have more knowledge and understanding of, people who are most similar to us. This is true in our lives as well as in our work, including in regard to the major variables of gender, race, ethnicity, ability, and social class (APA, 2003). Most of us are more comfortable providing services to people about whom we know most about, and often they are people most similar to us. Unfortunately, we also have a tendency to not only avoid but also to feel anxiety, fear, and/or anger toward those different from us. To practice ethically requires that we be aware of and manage and rise above those reactions through our cognitive and emotional skills so that we can provide sensitivity and empathy for the client as an individual.

All mental health associations provide various principles and standards that articulate professional expectations, including about therapists' work with diverse populations, based partly on the knowledge that it may take special effort to become prepared to work with those different from us. APA's (2017a) *Ethical Principles of Psychologists and Code of Conduct* includes such standards. The principles include the mandate that we respect the dignity and worth of each individual; that we are aware enough not to engage in unfair, discriminatory, and harassing or demeaning behaviors; and that we maintain evidence-based knowledge about the groups with whom we work.

The specific standard relevant to multicultural competence is the APA (2017a) Ethics Code (Standard 2.01, Boundaries of Competence):

(a) Psychologists provide services, teach, and conduct research with populations and in areas only within the boundaries of their competence, based on their education, training, supervised experience, consultation, study, or professional experience.

(b) Where scientific or professional knowledge in the discipline of psychology establishes that an understanding of factors associated with age, gender, gender identity, race, ethnicity, culture, national origin, religion, sexual orientation, disability, language, or socioeconomic status is essential for effective implementation of their services or research, psychologists have or obtain the training, experience, consultation, or supervision necessary to ensure the competence of their services, or they make appropriate referrals, except as provided in Standard 2.02, Providing Services in Emergencies.

In the APA, several special guidelines have been developed to provide more specific guidance for providers who work with members of diverse populations, including but not limited to the following:

- *Multicultural Guidelines: An Ecological Approach to Context, Identity, and Intersectionality* (APA, 2017b; https://www.apa.org/about/policy/multicultural-guidelines.pdf)
- *APA Guidelines for Psychological Practice With Girls and Women* (APA, 2018b; https://www.apa.org/about/policy/psychological-practice-girls-women.pdf)

- *Guidelines for Psychological Practice With Lesbian, Gay, and Bisexual Clients* (APA, 2012; https://www.apa.org/pubs/journals/features/amp-a0024659.pdf)
- *Guidelines for Psychological Practice With Older Adults* (APA, 2014b; https://www.apa.org/pubs/journals/features/older-adults.pdf)
- *Guidelines for Assessment of and Intervention With Persons With Disabilities* (APA, 2011a; https://www.apa.org/pi/disability/resources/assessment-disabilities)
- *APA Guidelines for Psychological Practice With Boys and Men* (APA, 2018a; https://www.apa.org/about/policy/boys-men-practice-guidelines.pdf)
- *Guidelines for Psychological Practice With Transgender and Gender Nonconforming People* (APA, 2015a; https://www.apa.org/practice/guidelines/transgender.pdf)
- *APA Guidelines for Psychological Practice for People With Low-Income and Economic Marginalization* (APA, 2019a; https://www.apa.org/about/policy/guidelines-low-income.pdf)
- *APA Guidelines on Race and Ethnicity in Psychology: Promoting Responsiveness and Equity* (APA, 2019b; https://www.apa.org/about/policy/guidelines-race-ethnicity.pdf)

Furthermore, the American Psychiatric Association's (2013) *Diagnostic and Statistical Manual of Mental Disorders* (5th ed.; *DSM-5*) addresses the importance of cultural variables in diagnosing mental disorders. Paniagua (2018) noted that the *DSM-5* advises mental health professionals against making diagnoses without considering cultural variables that might explain presenting symptoms. He also drew attention to the fact that although the World Health Organization's (WHO's; 1993) *International Classification of Diseases* (10th ed.; *ICD-10*) is normed across diverse WHO countries, it does not alert mental health practitioners to the need to pay attention to cultural variables before diagnosing people with mental disorders.

In 2013, the American Psychiatric Association and *DSM-5* began offering the Cultural Formulation Interview (CFI) to facilitate clinical understanding and decision making. Its Informant Version (there are also questions for the Interviewer) assesses issues such as sources of help (e.g., folk healing, religious or spiritual counseling), most salient elements of the individual's cultural identity (e.g., migration problems, conflict across generations or due to gender roles), and concerns about the clinician-patient relationship (e.g., perceptions of bias, communication barriers, or identity differences that may undermine effective delivery of service).

OVERVIEW

This monograph is designed to provide an overview of multicultural therapy. Chapter 2 describes a brief history and development of ethnic minority psychology to provide a context for understanding the evolution of this important approach to psychotherapy. This history provides the necessary background to understanding the foundation upon which contemporary theory and applications have been built.

The theory, goals, and key concepts of multicultural psychotherapy are presented in Chapter 3, including a description of the general principles that underlie activities related to the delivery of competent services to diverse populations. One of the goals of the chapter is to promote an understanding of the influence of the contextual and systemic factors (e.g., cultural, community) on the client as well as on the psychotherapist. Not only do they affect human development, including how one copes with life's challenges, but those factors also influence the process of psychotherapy. The three overarching factors of awareness, knowledge, and skills are expounded to promote multicultural competency.

The processes involved in the primary change mechanisms involved in multicultural therapy are described in Chapter 4. What are universal approaches to therapy versus culturally specific approaches relevant in each case? Various issues are addressed, such as the therapist–client relationship, the role of the therapist, and the role of the client. Strategies and techniques such as identification of areas of strengths and weaknesses and cultural adaptations of various evidence-based practices are propounded. A longer case study is provided in an attempt to illustrate some of the suggested strategies, while unique issues in the assessment process are also briefly addressed.

Chapter 5 provides evidence that multiculturalism has been integrated into the three foundational theoretical orientations of psychodynamic, humanistic, and cognitive behaviorism. Evaluation of multicultural therapy, including the identification of points of congruence and areas of differences between multicultural therapy and other orientations, is described. This chapter allows the reader to more thoroughly understand the importance and relevance of culture in their treatment approaches. In this chapter, we also strongly propose that social justice is an integral aspect of multiculturalism and argue that competent multicultural therapists include social justice work as part of an ethical practice.

Because the promotion of multicultural competence is such an important, lifelong developmental process, we include a chapter on education, training, and professional development. Chapter 6 provides an overview of how education and training, licensing, and continuing education have attended to and addressed multiculturalism and diversity in psychology.

Finally, Chapter 7 summarizes the major thrusts of the book and emphasizes the importance of social justice as part of the foundation of competent and ethical multicultural therapy. Issues for the future development of multicultural therapy are also considered.

2

History

The publication of *Multiculturalism as a Fourth Force* (Pedersen, 1999a) is considered by scholars in the counseling and psychotherapy fields to be a milestone in the history of psychology (Pedersen et al., 2016). The contribution examined the prospect that we are moving toward a universal theory of multiculturalism that recognizes the psychological consequences of each cultural context, where each behavior has been learned and is demonstrated. The term *fourth force* emphasizes that multiculturalism is relevant throughout the field of psychology as a generic rather than an exotic perspective (Pedersen, 1999b) and contextualizes it within the evolution of psychological theories and practice.

Many thought leaders of the field (e.g., Bernal et al., 2003; Carlson & Englar-Carlson, 2010; Pedersen, 2002; S. Sue, 1998) describe multiculturalism as a "fourth force," or fourth dimension of psychology that builds upon the three prior classical dimensions of psychological theory and scholarship marking the discipline: psychodynamic, behavioral, and

https://doi.org/10.1037/0000279-002
Multicultural Therapy: A Practice Imperative, by M. J. T. Vasquez and J. D. Johnson
Copyright © 2022 by the American Psychological Association. All rights reserved.

humanistic psychologies. This new wave recognizes the psychological implications of identities and contexts and calls attention to the way in which a culture-centered lens influences the way we perceive psychology across fields and theories (Pedersen, 1999a). Many theorists have incorporated multiculturalism in their models. Wampold and Imel (2015), for example, expanded social context to their conceptualization of psychotherapy effectiveness in their second edition of *The Great Psychotherapy Debate: The Evidence for What Makes Psychotherapy Work.*

In their introduction to the fifth edition of *Counseling Across Cultures*, Pedersen et al. (2002) described how their first edition was generally recognized as one of the earliest of a number of comprehensive books addressing the problems facing multicultural counseling. They described how the idea of the book evolved from a 1973 meeting of the American Psychological Association (APA) held in Montreal, where seven psychologists participated in a symposium by the same name as the book, *Counseling Across Cultures*. The papers were developed into a book that was published in 1976 by University of Hawaii Press as a monograph. That first edition went through five printings. By the time of its seventh edition (Lonner et al., 2016), multicultural awareness in all counseling relationships was perceived to be the rule rather than the exception. In addition, various aspects of identity, including gender, age, ability status, sexual orientation, immigration status, and others, were identified as having "culture" and were considered important identity variables to attend to in addition to race, ethnicity, and culture.

Multicultural theory in counseling and psychotherapy is based on the development of multicultural psychology. What is *multicultural psychology*? Mio et al. (2009) defined it as "the systematic study of behavior, cognition, and affect in settings where people of different backgrounds interact" (p. 3). It is the examination of the effect of culture on the way people act, think, and feel. Multicultural psychology assumes that it is impossible to understand any psychological processes without understanding the context in which they are embedded (La Roche, 2013). Culture is an "external factor" because it informs the events that occur around us and our interactions with other people, but culture also influences our internal processes, such as how we interpret the things around us (Mio et al., 2009). Multicultural psychotherapy, therefore, emphasizes the importance of using cultural information to more fully and accurately understand our clients and develop effective interventions.

Other terms used to define multicultural psychology include cultural psychotherapy (La Roche, 2013), cross-cultural psychotherapy and counseling (Marsella & Pedersen, 1980), ethnicity and family therapy (McGoldrick et al., 2005), multicultural counseling (D. W. Sue et al., 2007), and medical anthropology and cultural psychiatry (Kleinman, 1988).

HISTORY OF ETHNIC MINORITY PSYCHOLOGY

History is important. Franklin (2009) suggested that as we bask in the growth of a significant multicultural focus in psychology, it is appropriate to take measure of the journey. History is significantly relevant to the present position of ethnic minority psychologies and multiculturalism to the field; understanding it can help to prepare for future challenges and goals.

Holliday and Holmes (2003) identified four major themes as they described the history of ethnic minority psychology in the United States. The first theme represents the use of theories and data to support the myths of the legitimacy of White superiority and the inferiority, exploitation, discrimination, and dispossession of the United States' racial ethnic minorities; in other words, scientific racism. The second theme involved the evolution of the challenge and critique of those negative, stereotypic notions. The third theme involved the pursuit of ethnic minority inclusion and participation in psychology's scientific and professional associations and literature. The fourth theme has been the development and promulgation of theories and interventions reflecting cultures, values, worldviews, and historical experiences of ethnic minority people.

The Myth of White Superiority

The first theme, using theory and science to support the myth of the legitimacy of White superiority, was described poignantly in Guthrie's (1976,

1998) *Even the Rat Was White: A Historical View of Psychology.* He described how ethnic minority psychologists were virtually nonexistent until the 1930s, when the first African American students began to enter graduate programs in psychology. The early roots of multicultural psychology consisted of research on racial group differences, and many of those efforts resulted in racist methodologies and conclusions. For example, Guthrie described the instruments used by psychologists and anthropologists to measure skin color, hair texture, thickness of lips, and other anthropomorphic investigations of racial differences, mental abilities, and character traits among the peoples of the world, especially people of African and Mexican origins. He also described the eugenics movement, which aimed to "improve" the genetic physical and mental composition of future generations. In addition to within the United States (Cohen, 2016), efforts aimed at "race betterment" were practiced in other countries, most notably in Germany with Hitler's efforts to create a "master race" (Deutsch, 2019).

Challenges to and Research on Effects of Racism

The second theme described by Holliday and Holmes (2003) emerged when early scholars, such as George I. Sánchez and Horace Mann Bond, criticized psychological, intellectual, and educational testing and psychometric studies that claimed mental inferiority of Mexican American and African American children and adults (Guthrie, 1976). They each provided those critiques in the late 1950s and 1960s (Romo, 1986; White, 2007). In addition, research by ethnic minority psychologists and allies began to focus on the effects of racism, discrimination, and poverty on individuals from ethnic minority backgrounds. Studies by Kenneth and Mamie Clark in 1939, for example, found that African American children tended to attribute more positive characteristics to White dolls or pictures versus Black dolls or pictures, when they were given an option to choose. They concluded that those responses indicated low self-esteem of African American children resulting from segregation, racism, and discrimination. The U.S. Supreme Court found the Clarks' work on the harmful effects of segregation to be so compelling that they cited it in their 1954 decision, *Brown v. Board of Education.*

Increased Presence of Ethnic Minority Psychologists

Brought on by the civil rights era of the 1950s through the 1970s, the third theme of ethnic minority psychology in the United States involved the growth and inclusion of ethnic minority students in institutions of higher education, overturning decades of educational disenfranchisement (Holliday, 2009). As a result, the number of students of color admitted to psychology graduate programs in the 1970s and 1980s was sufficiently large to constitute a cohort. This group of ethnic minority psychologists was "confronted with the challenges of establishing a place in psychology's occupational and organizational structures, collegial networks, securing an intellectual space with psychology, and acquiring sufficient authority to make a difference" (Holliday, 2009, p. 317). During this time, the emergence of research and theoretical development among ethnic minority psychologists began to focus on the effects of racism, discrimination, and poverty on individuals from racial and ethnic minority backgrounds (Mio et al., 2009).

Development and Promulgation of Ethnic Minority Psychological Literature

The fourth theme described by Holliday and Holmes (2003) involves the development and promulgation of theories and interventions reflecting cultures, values, worldviews, and historical experiences of ethnic minority people. The paradigm of intersectionality is an important aspect of this fourth theme because the ways in which individuals are shaped by and identify with racial, ethnic, cultural, gender, sexual orientation, educational, economic, and social states are multitudinous and unique. Intersectionality lenses in psychology honor the complexities of our humanity as we navigate multiple dimensions of our identities within sociopolitical power statuses that create our lived experiences.

OTHER INFLUENCES OF THE DEVELOPMENT OF ETHNIC MINORITY PSYCHOLOGY

A "snapshot" of the history and development of ethnic minority psychology was provided in a special issue of *Cultural Diversity and Ethnic Minority Psychology*, the official journal of the APA's Division 45, Society of the Psychological Study of Ethnic Minority Issues (now named Society for the Psychological Study of Culture, Ethnicity and Race; Leong, 2009). Holliday (2009) presented a history of African American psychology; Trimble and Clearing-Sky (2009) provided a profile of American Indians and Alaska Natives in psychology; Leong and Okazaki (2009) wrote of the history of Asian Americans in psychology; Padilla and Olmedo (2009) contributed a synopsis of key persons, events, and associations in the history of Latinx psychology; and McCubbin and Marsella (2009) provided a cultural and historical context of Native Hawaiians. S. Sue's (2009) reflection on the history of ethnic minority psychology included the view that despite significant diversity among and within every ethnic group, there are striking similarities, including (a) that underrepresentation existed in the number of psychologists from each ethnic minority group, which had significant effects on the field; (b) a dearth of research, theory, and knowledge existed about the ethnic groups; (c) the available knowledge was based on biased, stereotypic, and racist assumptions; and (d) many practices in psychology failed to promote the welfare of ethnic minority groups. S. Sue (2009) also noted that the pioneers described in each of the ethnic groups were "extraordinary, ordinary people" who were neither privileged nor who came from severely impoverished backgrounds (p. 412). S. Sue (2009) identified four characteristics common among the pioneering leaders of each described group, including courage, intolerance of injustice, finding ways to significantly contribute, and commitment to ethnic/cultural/racial concerns.

The articles in the special issue described the long and complex history of race and ethnicity brimming with racism and various forms of oppression, including physical, social, and intellectual. They also described themes for the various groups discussed in regard to the centrality of culture, history, and pride in resilience (Franklin, 2009). In addition to describing how people of color were treated historically in the United States, descriptions were provided of how they were represented in the psychological literature. With the bias in society reflected within psychology, the implications for training, research, and practice were profound, creating unique challenges for ethnic minority psychologists, their professional organizations, and the movement of multicultural psychology in general (Franklin, 2009).

Various conferences and key events contributed to the expansion of roles of ethnic minority groups in psychology and within the APA. S. Sue (2009) noted that The Dulles Conference (in 1978), convened by Dalmas Taylor and James Jones, was the foundation for the establishment of the APA Office of Ethnic Minority Affairs (in 1979), the Board of Ethnic Minority Affairs (in 1980), the Society for the Psychological Study of Ethnic Minority Issues (in 1986), and the National Multicultural Conference and Summit (in 1999). Despite initial contentiousness about intersectional representation, principles of equity in representation from various groups were strongly voiced and supported, which has led to a strong sense of fellowship, collegiality, enthusiasm, and mutual support among different ethnic minority groups in the evolution of various structures of the APA, including the founding of the Public Interest Directorate (S. Sue, 2009).

The increased focus on multiculturalism in psychology was described by Franklin (2009) as a natural outgrowth of our independent and collaborative work via ethnic psychological associations. Today they include the American Black Psychological Association, the National Latinx Psychological Association, the Asian American Psychological Association, the Society of Indian Psychologists, and, more recently, the Middle Eastern, North African Psychological Association. Franklin also credited a variety of allies and a new cadre of colleagues within the general membership of the APA. He noted, for example, APA Division 9, Society for the Psychological Study of Social Issues, for their focus on human rights and social justice and as an early supporter of inclusion and advocacy for ethnic minority psychology. Division 17, Society of Counseling Psychology, emerged over several decades as a major leader for multicultural counseling and inclusion of multiculturalism into training, research, and practice. Furthermore, diversity became the thematic priority at the foundation of APA Divisions 35 (Society for Psychology of Women), 44 (Society for the Psychology of Sexual Orientation and Gender Diversity), and 45 (Society for the Psychological Study of Culture, Ethnicity and Race).

Franklin (2009) suggested that a significant theme in the origins of ethnic minority psychology is the centrality of culture, history, and pride in our resilience as a people. The history described in that special issue contained a passionate recounting of the deeply scarring indignities experienced due to discrimination and pejorative treatment as ethnic minorities in the United States. He also noted that a catalyst for confronting the profession of psychology was a reaction to historic deficit orientations for ethnic minorities in the literature and research, and that the challenges the ethnic psychological associations undertook to redress the failings of the field were a direct result of the pressing need to transform the status quo in the profession.

The evolution of "empirically supported treatments" (ESTs) in the 1990s was considered to have had substantial impact in psychology, particularly for the validation of procedures for specific psychological problems (Tolin et al., 2015). However, the failure of ESTs to include and examine different racial/ethnic populations was problematic. With ESTs, there was no clear way to establish whether a treatment had proven effective with diverse populations. There has also been the recognition that patients may be more complex or heterogeneous than those in efficacy-oriented randomized controlled trials (Tolin et al., 2015). Thus, an American Psychological Association Presidential Task Force produced a report that helped establish policy in APA for evidence-based practice in psychology (EBPP). In an integration of science and practice, the policy took into account the full range of evidence that psychologists and policymakers must consider, including research findings, clinical expertise, and patient characteristics. These are all considered as relevant to good outcomes (APA Task Force on Evidence-Based Practice, 2006). Thus, there was recognition that cultural factors, such as those within patient and research participant characteristics, and clinical expertise, that includes multicultural competence, were important factors to consider in treatment planning and implementation.

The historic failings in psychology, including the negative and painful treatment of racial/ethnic groups in psychological research as described by Guthrie (1976, 1998), as well as the invisibility of racial/ethnic groups in the evolution of research methodologies such as ESTs, have negatively influenced the development of theory, research, and training of applied psychology and psychotherapy practice. Fortunately, many practitioners and researchers who study practice and therapeutic interventions have worked hard to promote more relevant and applicable approaches to the development of effective and meaningful interventions for diverse groups. In the next chapter, we address the theory, goals, and key concepts of multi-cultural therapy.

3

Theory, Goals, and Key Concepts

As described briefly in the Introduction and elaborated further in this chapter, the theory of multicultural therapy involves the description of how competence is developed within the context of three overarching domains that define the multiculturally competent psychotherapist: awareness, knowledge, and skills. They are thus goals in the ongoing quest to gain and maintain the competence that includes understanding the influence of cultures, contexts, and systemic issues on clients and therapists as well as on the process and outcome of therapy. To enhance the probability that psychotherapists attend to multicultural dynamics within the therapeutic relationship and provide effective treatment for racial and ethnic minority clients, they must develop awareness, knowledge, and skills regarding the cultural and identity issues presented in the context of the therapeutic relationship.

https://doi.org/10.1037/0000279-003
Multicultural Therapy: A Practice Imperative, by M. J. T. Vasquez and J. D. Johnson

This chapter provides more detail involving key concepts in the development of these three domains. We draw from the social psychological literature as well as the various multicultural approaches and worldviews that have been developed and discussed, with the belief that obtaining cultural awareness, enhancing cultural knowledge, and developing culturally responsive skills and interventions contributes to multicultural competence and effectiveness. The processes are complex. They may involve multicultural learning experiences that are developmentally professionally appropriate that build on levels of psychotherapist competence from student–trainee to proficient professional. Our goal is to provide information and direction to contribute to those processes.

AWARENESS

Acquiring multicultural awareness is an ongoing goal. This has to do with metacognitive awareness of one's attitudes and beliefs that influence behavioral responses to others as well as awareness of others' experiences in life and the development of their attitudes, beliefs, and behaviors. For example, one critical area of awareness has to do with the question of how various identities and social locations—*social location* being the social position a person holds within society based on characteristics and qualities deemed to be important by any given society, including gender, social class, race, education, abilities, and age—shape experiences and outcomes. Failure to develop an awareness of how social-political categories depend on one another for meaning renders knowledge of any one category both incomplete and possibly biased. Attending to a client's various social-political categories can increase awareness and lead to a more nuanced understanding of how identity, difference, privilege, and disadvantage shape experiences and influence people's relationships, their responses to various elements in society, and the responses of others to them as well. Cole (2009) described how categories such as race, gender, social class, and sexual identity do not simply describe groups that may be different or similar, they also encapsulate complex historical and ongoing political, material, and social disparities and stigma. Understanding the interplay between person and social location, with particular emphasis on power relations among various social locations, is part of the goal of becoming multiculturally competent (Cole, 2009; Mahalingam, 2007).

Assisting and encouraging psychotherapists to become self-aware and to examine their cultural attitudes and beliefs is an important goal in developing multicultural competence and increasing counselor effectiveness with culturally diverse clients. D. W. Sue and Sue (2013) conceptualized the importance of developing awareness through self-examination of attitudes, beliefs, and feelings associated with cultural differences.

Additionally, developing awareness of the experiences of the culturally diverse clients with whom we work helps shape our attitudes, our empathy, and our way of being with diverse clients. Awareness facilitates emotional concern about the particular experiences of the individuals with whom we work. It increases our ability to have *cultural empathy*, that is, empathy based on well-informed interest of as much of the identities and experiences of the persons with whom we work. The following sections describe specific areas we deem important to promote those awarenesses and related qualities that contribute to multicultural therapy competence.

Awareness of Barriers to Effective Treatment of Multicultural Clients

Ethnic minority populations underutilize psychotherapy services and have high rates of dropping out of treatment (McGuire & Miranda, 2008). Racial disparities were found in both the types of treatment received (e.g., psychotherapy and medications for major depressive disorder) and the length of treatment over the decade examined by Connolly Gibbons et al. (2011). For example, findings from a database of approximately 300,000 public sector clients in 2003 demonstrated that White people received significantly more psychotherapy sessions than 10 years earlier, receiving an average of 15 sessions in 2003 versus 10 in 1993. In comparison, African Americans in the same database received far fewer psychotherapy appointments on average in 1993 and had a significantly smaller increase in the number of psychotherapy sessions attended over the decade, with an average of only nine in 2003.

Another barrier to effective treatment may be the differential effects of psychotropic medications on various racial and ethnic minority people. For example, Chaudhry et al. (2008) reviewed the literature on the role of race and ethnicity in psychopharmacology and reported findings of ethnic differences in clinical presentation, treatment, and response. They cited studies demonstrating that African American patients diagnosed with bipolar disorder needed lower doses of lithium treatment because higher doses resulted in increased side effects. Chaudhry et al. further showed that, compared with White Americans, Asian Americans have a lower threshold for therapeutic and adverse effects with antipsychotic drugs. They also cited data that found that in comparison with White American women, Hispanic American women complained about common side effects when given half the dose of tricyclic antidepressants. Chaudhry et al. concluded that when ethnicity is "defined based upon shared genetic and cultural/environmental background, it is clear that ethnicity is indeed an important influence on psychotropic drug response" (p. 678).

In another study, Wu et al. (2012) used the Market Scan Multi-State Medicaid Database to examine a total of 3,038 Medicaid enrollees diagnosed with major depressive disorder and comorbid anxiety. They found that although African Americans were significantly less likely to have office visits related to mental health than White Americans, they were more likely to go to the emergency department and be hospitalized for the same conditions. The authors concluded that disparities in mental health care use between African and White Americans still exist.

Multiple reasons most likely account for the findings in less utilization of mental health services, such as lack of health insurance and out-of-pocket costs of services, disparities in access to resources, and stigma about the use of mental health services; these are all issues that must be addressed at a societal level. An additional possibility may be that many ethnic minority clients do not experience a beneficial therapeutic alliance, partly due to cultural misunderstandings and miscommunications between psychotherapists and their clients. We may not always be aware of when the potential for developing an effective therapeutic alliance may be compromised. For example, Hill et al. (1993) suggested that clients may have a tendency to defer and conceal negative reactions within the therapeutic relationship and that we should create opportunities for clients to express themselves more authentically. Although disguising negative emotions is a natural human process (Hill et al., 1993), clients may hide their reactions out of fear of rejection if they express negative feelings to their therapist, and/or out of deference to the therapist's authority.

Premature termination is a major barrier to successful treatment outcomes regardless of theoretical orientation (M. B. C. Gibbons et al., 2019; King & Boswell, 2019), disorder (Philips et al., 2018; Swift & Greenberg, 2014), or place of service (Sharf et al., 2010; Xiao et al., 2017). The issue is particularly significant when race and ethnicity are variables. In examining archival data, Kilmer et al. (2019) found that racial/ethnic minority (REM) clients were more likely to terminate after a single session than non-REM clients. They suggested "greater emphasis on integrating multicultural competencies in work with clients" (p. 94). This may help in mitigating early termination. When premature termination of psychotherapy was examined in connection with therapeutic alliance, cultural competence, and minority status, Anderson et al. (2019) found that it was associated with therapists who were perceived to have low multicultural competence.

Awareness of the Importance of and Threats to the Therapeutic Alliance

The therapeutic alliance is one of the most important aspects of therapeutic effectiveness (Hill & Williams, 2000). However, many, if not most, people of color encounter microaggressions so frequently that they have developed a coping strategy to "edit" their responses on a regular basis. This response, combined with cultural values, may further inhibit the expression of negative reactions. Therefore, it is helpful to be aware of a client's negative reactions that interfere with the development of a positive alliance or even cause alliance ruptures. A helpful strategy might be to check in with them about reactions to challenges, interpretations, and suggestions, for example, "I can't get everything right, and I may miss the boat on big and small things. But I want to be helpful. Therefore, I invite you to share with me your feedback, thoughts, and feelings about what's going on in here."

Although there is mixed evidence, most clients of color are more comfortably matched with therapists like themselves (Casas et al., 2002; Pedersen et al., 2002; D. W. Sue & Sue, 2003). More specifically, clients working with clinicians of similar ethnic backgrounds and languages tend to remain in treatment longer than do clients whose therapists are neither ethnically nor linguistically matched (D. W. Sue & Sue, 2003). Unfortunately, such matches are not always possible or even desired. Swift et al. (2015) found that clients in psychotherapy preferred that therapists have multicultural training and use culturally adapted treatments to racial/ ethnic matching. Further, Rodriguez et al. (2008) cautioned that similarities can mask important cultural snares for the therapist. Cabral and Smith (2011) conducted a meta-analysis of racial/ethnic matching research and concluded that there is a great deal of variability in results.

Our worldviews are influenced in large part by our cultural backgrounds, including the way we view our lives and our experiences, as well as those of others. As cultural beings, we all have conscious and subconscious schemata that inform our interactions with others in the various areas of our lives, including in our professional work. We are all vulnerable to implicit bias, and the social psychological literature indicates that even those of us holding egalitarian beliefs behave in discriminatory ways to those who are different from us (Allport, 1954; Dovidio et al., 2002; Greenwald & Banaji, 1995; Opotow, 1990; D. W. Sue & Sue, 2003). Specifically, our societal structures have compounding effects on our cognitive schemata, and consequently our attitudes and beliefs about people. The way cultural images of groups are formed influences the social order and has considerable effect on the identities of people in various groups, both ethnic minority and White majority. Such representations have an impact on our implicit judgments of, and behaviors toward, others (Greenwald & Banaji, 1995). Because these processes are frequently hidden in the subconscious, mental health providers may not always be aware of when the establishment of an effective therapeutic alliance is being undermined by their or their clients' attitudes and beliefs about themselves and each other. We could thus unwittingly compromise the cultural sensitivity and cultural empathy that Tseng and Streltzer (2004) described as essential to be a culturally competent clinician.

As noted previously, the automatic assumptions underlying stereotypes and generalizations, and their corresponding behaviors, are typically subconscious; we often are not made aware of them until someone calls them to our attention. No one is immune to these processes, including ethnic minority psychologists, even toward our own ethnic group members. Living in a society that continuously demeans images of one's identity group, negative internalization of racism can occur; this is a phenomenon that is important for the practitioner to understand as well. "Internalized racism" can be subtle, unconscious, and powerfully destructive, and we must all work toward eradicating it within ourselves and each other (Cross, 1971).

It is thus important for providers of therapeutic services to maintain knowledge of the evidence-based information about language and behaviors considered demeaning to those from different groups and to continuously develop awareness of one's biases about groups of people who are systematically devalued in society. Subconsciously, we may be affected by the fact that an identity group of someone we work with is beyond our personal and professional experience, increasing the chances that our treatment may be compromised. Similarly, providers need to be aware of the impact of biases presumed to be positive. For example, Atkin et al. (2018) reported that internalizing the stereotype of the "model minority," which assumes unrestricted upward socioeconomic and educational mobility, increases depression and anxiety among Asian American adolescents. As clinicians, we need to be cautious about these beliefs as well.

To illustrate, Dr. V saw a new client with a heavy Spanish accent. Because of the accent, I assumed that her employment at her company was as clerical staff. In the first session, I learned that not only was she an administrator in her work setting, but she was also highly credentialed, effective, and involved in training other administrators. I was aware of the appreciation and admiration I felt for her, and I simultaneously felt frustrated by my own vulnerability to being influenced by perceived status variables, the one I assumed and the one that was real. After all, shouldn't we regard all of our clients and all of their employment positions as deserving of respect and consideration? We believe that, but the fact is that we are all influenced by multiple variables. The point is to try to be as aware as possible when some of those influences come from our biases, and make efforts to correct them.

Awareness of Categorization: Constructive and Destructive Strategy

One of the things we do when we perceive others is to place them in a category. This well-documented psychological process helps us organize overwhelming amounts of information to reduce it into manageable chunks that go together (Allport, 1954). When this normal cognitive process leads us to associating certain traits and behaviors with particular groups, even if they are factually not generalizable for most individuals within those groups, stereotyping is the consequence. In addition to constructing personal narratives, these categories (e.g., race, gender) provide instantaneous explanations of how life works and signify differential power and value (Walker, 2020).

Furthermore, we subconsciously automatically create "us versus them" dichotomies (Jamieson et al., 2013; Opotow, 1990), categorizing people into *ingroups*, those with whom we identify, and *outgroups*, those from whom we deidentify. We value, trust, and cooperate more with people we perceive as being in our "ingroup" as opposed to people we perceive as being "them." We also have more compassion for, and are more likely to endorse and support, people in our ingroup than those people we perceive as being in outgroups.

When entire communities identify others as being in an outgroup, they implicitly conceptualize those outgroup members as "them," and these categorizations affect behaviors of individuals in both groups. We tend to objectify outgroup members, behaving toward them in insensitive ways. At minimum, we ignore or neglect them, but as history has proven, these behaviors can extend to the point of engaging in hate crimes and genocidal activities.

According to FBI statistics, almost 60% of hate crimes in the last few years were motivated by race, ethnicity, or ancestry bias (U.S. Department of Justice, Federal Bureau of Investigation, 2016). Other diverse identities, such as sexual orientation, also evoke shockingly destructive behaviors. Specific horrific examples of hate crimes include the murders in 1998 of Matthew Shepard, a gay man in Wyoming, and of James Byrd, Jr., an African American in Texas; both deaths brought national and international attention and a movement to enact hate-crime legislation at the state and federal levels. These two atrocious crimes compelled members of Congress to pass the Matthew Shepard and James Byrd, Jr., Hate Crimes Prevention Act of 2009 (HCPA P. L. No. 111–84), which extended the FBI's investigative scope into crimes not only restricted to those wherein the victim was engaged in a federally protected activity, it also authorized investigations of hate crimes beyond the victim's race, color, religion, or national origin by including those crimes that were based on actual or perceived sexual orientation, gender identity, and disability.

The COVID-19 pandemic, first reported in the city of Wuhan, Hubei, China, in December 2019, led to a worldwide increase in acts of hate crimes and displays of prejudice, xenophobia, and racism against people of East Asian, North Asian, and Southeast Asian descent. Groups such as the Asian American Psychological Association supported the COVID-19 Hate Crimes Act (Pub. L. 117-13), which would allow the U.S. Justice Department to review hate crimes related to COVID-19 and establish an online database. It received bipartisan support in the U.S. House and Senate and was signed into law by President Biden on May 20, 2021.

In the past few decades, there has been unprecedented public outcry over unarmed Black men, women, and children brutalized or killed by police and other self-proclaimed "watch" persons. Trayvon Martin was a young African American man who was killed while walking in his father's predominantly White neighborhood. He was stopped, questioned, and killed by a self-proclaimed neighborhood watchman, George Zimmerman, who apparently believed that Black teenagers engage in robbery and saw Trayvon Martin as part of an outgroup. The complex individual biases and negative societal constructions of race and ethnicity have led to many tragic police-involved deaths of people of color, especially

Black and Brown men, women, and children. Fear and anxiety are underlying emotions related to interactions between those in power and people of color. Ta-Nehisi Coates authored an award-winning book that consists of a letter to his son. In it, he wrote that one of his friends, killed by a police officer, "was not killed by a single officer so much as he was killed by his country and all the fears that have marked it from birth" (Coates, 2015, p. 77). Popular writings such as that of Coates hopefully increase understanding of these complex problems within the general population.

With the advent of social media, several other horrific events have been made public, including the brutal murder of another African American man, George Floyd, by a police officer who kept his knee on Mr. Floyd's neck for more than 9 minutes, despite the fact that Mr. Floyd kept saying, "I can't breathe," and despite bystanders' pleas to the police officer to let up (Bennett et al., 2020). This murder, fortunately recorded and publicized, led to an unparalleled outcry heard around the world and is described in more detail at the end of Chapter 5, in the section titled Social Justice. It is estimated that as of early July 2020, the millions of demonstrators, including people from a diverse group of races and ethnicities in the United States, constituted the largest protests in U.S. history ("How George Floyd's Death," 2020).

The effects of negative categorizations are significant. Researchers (e.g., Jamieson et al., 2013; Mendes et al., 2007; Shamsudheen, 2013) have found that people are more sensitive to experiences of discrimination perpetuated against them by people outside of their group than by people within their group. Feelings of threat and shame result from ingroup discrimination, whereas discrimination by outgroup members instigates anger due to perceptions of being challenged. When we experience discrimination from those whom we perceive to be like us, our cortisol levels tend to increase, we experience impairments in our short-term memory, and there are increases in vascular resistance; collectively, these effects have been shown to lead to cognitive impairments if discrimination is experienced chronically (Shamsudheen, 2013). Jamieson et al. (2013) also found that people experiencing outgroup discrimination had feelings of anger, hypervigilance, and higher risk behaviors predisposing them to dangerous behaviors compared with people experiencing ingroup discrimination.

As demonstrated, categorization can have negative effects, but it can have positive benefits as well. A strategy of intervention is to emphasize positive role models from an individual's identity groups. Positive role models are reminders that exceptional people exist in all groups, particularly when they are provided with opportunities to apply their talents. When people such as U.S. Supreme Court Justice Sonia Sotomayor or President Barack Obama are appointed or elected to positions of power, it potentially evokes positive feelings about one's identity group. A family of color in the White House is certainly something that many of us never expected to see in our lifetimes. It was joyful to celebrate. Regardless of your political orientation, you must know that it was a psychologically powerful event in the lives of many Native American women when the first two Native American women to serve in the U.S. Congress— Congresswomen Sharice Davids (D-KS) and Deb Haaland (D-NM)— were both reelected and joined by a third, Yvette Herrell (R-NM), in 2021. Athletes, journalists, writers, entertainers, and other public figures who represent various diverse groups can have a positive impact on their identity group members as well as the general public. Think back to your reactions to someone highly visible or prominent who represented your identity group, for better or worse, and then think about how that made you feel about yourself. Helping clients think about positive role models in their everyday life, as well as in the media, can be a helpful strategy in promoting positive images of one's identity group.

Awareness of Contemporary Aversive Racism

Various studies have indicated that it is difficult, if not impossible, to be color-blind; as much as we perceive ourselves to be egalitarian, we are not subconsciously color-blind. Researchers and scholars (e.g., Dovidio et al., 2002, 2016) have demonstrated that contemporary racism among White individuals is subtle, often unintentional, and unconscious, but the consequences are systematically harmful. Racism promotes miscommunication and distrust.

These researchers found that White employers and admissions counselors exhibited less eye contact and their voice tones were not as warm or natural when interacting with people who were different from themselves (Dovidio et al., 2002, 2016). In their studies, although the White interviewers were not aware of the negative body language, the African American interviewees were very aware of it. Employee selection and promotion studies continuously find bias, especially when those behaviors can be based on some factor other than race (Dovidio et al., 2002, 2016; J. M. Jones, 1998). Plausible deniability is demonstrated by such attitudes as when potential employers in the academy describe that a female candidate is well published but has too few solo authored publications or that the journals she publishes in are not premiere journals. It is not considered or valued that women in academia may be more relational and mentor colleagues and students by coauthoring. These authors further demonstrated how "aversive racism," a form of individual-level prejudice characterizing the thoughts, feelings, and behaviors of the majority of well-intentioned and ostensibly nonprejudiced White Americans, contributes to the continued perpetuation of unfair racial disparities in the United States (Dovidio et al., 2016). For example, when employment applicants' credentials clearly qualified or disqualified them for a position, there was no discrimination against the Black candidate, but when the candidates' qualifications were more moderate, White participants selected the Black candidate significantly less often than the White candidate with exactly the same credentials (Dovidio et al., 2016).

Based on Dovidio et al.'s (2002) studies that indicate that ethnic minorities are aware of the disconnect projected by interviewers, it is important to realize that some, if not most, minority group members may be particularly sensitive to signs of rejection, dislike, or discrimination displayed unconsciously by the provider of services (Dovidio et al., 2002; Vasquez, 2007a, 2007b). It takes more energy and cognitive effort and flexibility on the part of the provider to attend to these issues.

In regard to "color-blindness," the stance that one takes when they state "I don't see color" or "We all bleed red" demonstrates that dominant-group members' diversity beliefs (e.g., multiculturalism, color-blindness) have palpable implications for minority colleagues' psychological engagement. Counterintuitively, focusing on reducing group differences reinforces majority privilege and minority marginalization (e.g., when "majority rule" meeting procedures are utilized). Whereas multiculturalism may promote inclusive behaviors and policies (Wolsko et al., 2006), color-blindness can perpetuate interpersonal and institutional discrimination through social distancing (Apfelbaum et al., 2008) and justification of inequality (Knowles et al., 2009; Saguy et al., 2008). Moreover, these findings converge with research showing that minorities are vigilant to inclusion-related cues and that color-blindness may signal bias (Apfelbaum et al., 2008; Purdie-Vaughns et al., 2008). Making multiple advances across areas of psychology, we have shown that poor diversity climates cost and positive diversity climates benefit both minorities and organizations.

It is thus important for each of us to be aware of the possibility of engaging in inappropriate, unconscious aversive racism. Pretending that one is "color-blind" and does not see race in their interactions promotes marginalization for someone who clearly knows their color is clear and not invisible. We may believe that we are open and accepting of all identity differences; however, our biases, preferences, and orientations are powerful influencers of our attitudes and behaviors—unless we work hard to make ourselves aware of them and work harder to eliminate them.

A Personal Example

Dr. V would like to share a personal experience about biases in the context of family and of religion. I would like to describe the experience of loss of my 83-year-old maternal grandmother, which will also illustrate the uniqueness of a Latinx death as well as my family's approach to death. My maternal grandmother was the last of my grandparents to die. Her husband, my grandfather, had died about 15 years before of a sudden heart attack. My grandmother had had a difficult time with it, but over time, she grew to enjoy her life again. A daughter or grand-daughter always lived with her, as is often the case in traditional Latinx families. Widowed Latinx mothers and grandmothers rarely live alone. My mother was the first-born in her family; I am the oldest grandchild. I had a nice, warm, and affectionate relationship with my grandmother; she had seven daughters, two sons, about 40 grandchildren, and several great-grandchildren.

When my grandmother was diagnosed with liver cancer at the age of 83, she chose not to receive treatment, which would have only extended her life a few weeks or months. Soon after she was diagnosed in the fall of that year, the family planned to have an early outdoor Thanksgiving feast at a small ranch owned by one of my uncles. It was a beautiful, cool, and sunny day, and some of the land had been cleared and prepared for us to bring lawn chairs, blankets, et cetera. Only immediate family and a few close old friends were invited; approximately 100 people were in attendance! The day began with an outdoor Catholic Mass. The majority of my aunts and uncles are Catholic. However, the uncle who hosted the event had married a Baptist woman and he had converted. After the Mass, they had their fundamentalist Baptist minister give a hellfire and damnation sermon in Spanish. Most of us politely watched from a distance and attempted not to roll our elitist, judgmental eyes. I admit, I was not religiously tolerant or respectful in that moment!

After the sermon, however, the Baptist minister asked that my grandmother, who was seated in a recliner under some trees, be surrounded by all nine of her sons and daughters. Then he had each, one at a time, kneel in front of her and say whatever it was that they needed to say before she died. The minister provided my grandmother with oil that she used to bless my mother, aunts, and uncles. The rest of us stood several yards away, out of earshot, in quiet respect as we observed the ritual, which took about 45 minutes. It was powerfully moving. That day, I witnessed the most effective and powerful resolution and closure activity! It was humbling to acknowledge that someone whom I had negatively appraised out of my unfamiliarity and negative bias had something so amazing to provide to this family in pain. The lesson was for me to be more respectful of what others have to offer. Even had he not conducted the ritual, his presence would have provided solace to some of my relatives, and I should have respected that.

My grandmother was expected to attend this event only for a couple of hours, as she was in fairly severe pain. Instead, she stayed for the whole day—about 8 hours! Her mood, and that of the entire group, was so warm, connected, and joyful that she seemed able to be present. She seemed to take in the love, respect, and care that was so lovingly given; there was an underlying sadness but also a sort of acceptance and an unspoken unity in being supportively present for her, and for each other! My grandmother sat under an open-air tent, and while my cousins played guitars, she sang songs of her childhood. Most of us, including some of her sons and daughters, learned just that day that she had traveled with her father, who was a minstrel of sorts, singing songs in various towns for money!

To this day, I feel incredibly fortunate to have experienced the events of that day. I learned a lesson, and I hope that I continue to not allow the distance that most of us automatically feel in response to that which is different or foreign to dictate my feelings, thoughts, and behaviors, in my personal life and especially in my professional work. My automatic assumption is that I would probably disagree with 90% or more of this fundamentalist minister's orientation to much of life, but after this experience, I find myself to be more open, more respectful despite differences, and appreciative that everyone has something to offer.

We have each had experiences where, most likely because of differences, our judgment and criticalness were misplaced, inappropriate, and unfounded. Is it ever OK to do so in the psychotherapy room, classroom, research labs, or organizations? On the other hand, how many times have you used your voice to intervene to support others? A recommended goal is to cultivate an attitude that predisposes us to finding the appreciation and value among people we perceive as different from us in the context of our work.

MULTICULTURAL KNOWLEDGE

Knowledge about diversity *within* social categories of identity, including disadvantages and privileges, can help therapists improve their ability to theorize and create treatment interventions to benefit members of those groups. To begin with, understanding and considering cultural issues are fundamental to professional behavior and practice. While there are many definitions of *cultural competence*, Tseng and Streltzer's (2004) definition is comprehensive and especially appropriate for mental health settings as it focuses on the impact of cultural issues in psychotherapy and other psychological applications. Per this definition, cultural competence is shown by the acquisition of three qualities and their service in the achievement of therapeutic goals.

The first quality is *cultural sensitivity*: knowledge and respect for culturally diverse people. We would add that this includes awareness and appreciation of one's cultural identity. This is the opposite of ethnocentricity, which sees differences as bad, negative, or less than, especially in comparison with one's own identity. For example, most racial and ethnic minority groups share values that promote a collective and family orientation, which is different from the Western, European individualistic, independent stance. Because the history of psychological theorists is populated by White European and American psychologists, our psychological theories tend to be influenced by those values. This has implications for our perceptions of clients who express values of connection to family, for example. The risk is to pathologize those individuals as "dependent" or incapable of "individuating."

The second quality is *cultural knowledge*, the factual information of fundamental anthropological knowledge about diversity within and between cultures. Cultural knowledge can be gained through classes, seminars, readings, professional consultations, and/or meaningful exchanges with culturally diverse individuals.

The third quality is *cultural empathy*, the ability to relate emotionally with the patient's cultural worldview. The culturally competent clinician provides what Tseng and Streltzer (2004) called cultural guidance: by determining whether and how the concerns a patient shares with us are linked to cultural factors and experiences and suggesting culturally appropriate therapeutic interventions to address those concerns. Increased awareness and experiences from working, socializing, living, and studying with people different from us leads to increased competence.

Whaley and Davis (2007) reviewed several definitions of cultural competence and found that all definitions concur that knowledge and skill proficiency relevant to the cultural background of the client is fundamental to said definition and that cultural perspective taking is an essential characteristic. In addition, the definition frequently includes organizational and system-level activities. Specifically, their definition is as follows:

> (a) the ability to recognize and understand the dynamic interplay between the heritage and adaptation dimensions of culture in shaping human behavior; (b) the ability to use the knowledge acquired about an individual's heritage and adaptational challenges to maximize the effectiveness of assessment, diagnosis, and treatment; and (c) internalization (i.e., incorporation into one's clinical problem-solving repertoire) of this process of recognition, acquisition, and use of cultural dynamics so that it can be routinely applied to diverse groups. (p. 565)

This definition is consistent with Tseng and Streltzer's (2004) in that a process model of cultural competence is less susceptible to cultural stereotypes than a content model, which stresses specific elements of culture for culturally different groups (Whaley & Davis, 2007).

Knowledge of Mental Health Disparities Among Racial and Ethnic Minority Populations

It's not enough to know that mental health disparities exist. The multiculturally competent therapist endeavors to understand why they exist to be effective in delivering appropriate prevention and intervention services that are accessible to the populations with whom they work. Studies of diverse populations can add to our understanding of risks for mental illness, responsiveness to prevention and treatment interventions, as well as access to, and engagement in, services. This information is essential to the development of specialized interventions. To this end, the availability of information about the mental health status of racial and ethnic minority populations is a priority for many organizations, including the National Institute on Minority Health and Health Disparities (NIMHD, 2020) of the National Institute of Mental Health (NIMH), and variations and disparities among and within these groups have been identified. NIMHD prioritizes research from genomics to services to detect and mitigate these disparities.

Several factors account for higher levels of psychological distress for various racial and ethnic minority populations. Poverty is one of the factors affecting mental health status for all people. For example, African Americans living below the poverty level are twice as likely to report psychological distress as compared with those above twice the poverty level (U.S. Department of Health and Human Services Office of Minority Health [USDHHS OMH], 2021a). Another factor is suicide, the second largest cause of death for African American young people aged 15 to 24 (USDHHS OMH, 2021a). The mortality rate for African American men in 2017 was 4 times higher than for African American women. And while for African Americans in general, the average suicide rate is 60% lower than for the non-Hispanic White population, alarmingly, African American girls in Grades 9 to 12 were 70% more likely to attempt suicide as compared with non-Hispanic White girls of the same age.

American Indians and Alaska Natives are twice as likely to experience feelings of nervousness or restlessness and twice as likely to experience the feeling that everything is an effort, all or most of the time, as compared with non-Hispanic Whites (USDHHS OMH, 2021b). American Indian and Alaska Native youth suffer disproportionately from death by suicide. In 2017, the rates of suicide were highest for American Indian and Alaska Native, non-Hispanic males (33.6 per 100,000) and females (11.0 per 100,000), followed by White, non-Hispanic males (28.2 per 100,000) and females (7.9 per 100,000; NIMH, 2017c). In 2017, suicide was the second leading cause of death for this population between the ages of 10 and 34 (USDHHS OMH, 2021b). Although the overall death rate for American Indians and Alaska Natives is comparable to that of the White population, adolescent American Indian and Alaska Native girls have death rates at almost 4 times the rate for White girls in the same age groups. Their causes of death include unintentional injuries, violence, or suicide. However, death rates can vary considerably among communities, even within the same region. Public health interventions and community efforts are being made to promote resilience and reduce the burden of causes of suicide among indigenous populations.

Although the causes of resilience among individuals and communities remain obscure, possible hypotheses include increased commitment to cultural values, spirituality, meaningful community involvement, and engagement in traditional activities. Culturally sensitive, public health approaches have yielded some successes, but it is not yet known what strategies are most effective to prevent suicide (NIMH, 2017a).

As it does in most other ethnic populations, the rate of serious psychological distress for Asian Americans increases with lower levels of income (USDHHS OMH, 2021c). Southeast Asian refugees are at risk for post-traumatic stress disorder (PTSD) associated with pre- and postimmigration trauma, with 70% of those receiving mental health care diagnosed with PTSD. While the prevalence of any mental illness reported is lowest for Asian adults (NIMH, 2017b), and the overall suicide rate for Asian Americans is half that of the White population, older Asian American women have the highest suicide rate of all women over age 65 in the United States (U.S. Department of Health & Human Services, 2001), and suicide was the leading cause of death for Asian Americans ages 15 to 24 in 2017. In fact, Asian American girls in Grades 9 through 12 were 20% more likely than non-Hispanic White girls to attempt suicide (USDHHS OMH, 2021c).

Hispanics living below the poverty level, as compared with Hispanics over twice the poverty level, are 3 times more likely to report psychological distress (USDHHS OMH, 2021d). While the suicide rate for Hispanics is less than half that of the non-Hispanic White population, like other racial and ethnic minorities, the suicide rates for Hispanic girls grades 9 through 12 were 40% higher than for non-Hispanic White girls in the same age group in 2017. Price and Khubchandani (2017) found that suicidal ideation and attempts were more prevalent among Latinx female adolescents than among White or African American youth. And while the suicide rate for Hispanic men was four times the rate for Hispanic women in 2017, non-Hispanic Whites received mental health treatment twice as often as Hispanics in 2018.

As noted above, health care quality and access are suboptimal for minority and low-income groups, and while overall quality is improving, access is getting worse, according to the *National Healthcare Quality and Disparities Report* (Agency for Healthcare Research and Quality, 2018). Access to mental health care is similarly disparate across race and ethnicity, geographic regions, and socioeconomic domains. Compared with the majority population, racial and ethnic minorities in the United States are less likely to have access to and to use mental health services, are more likely to use inpatient hospitalization and emergency departments, and are more likely to receive poorer quality of care (Substance Abuse and Mental Health Services Administration, 2015). For nearly every therapeutic intervention, ethnic minority Americans receive fewer procedures and poorer treatment than White Americans. Across all racial and ethnic groups, fees associated with treatments and lack of insurance was the most common reason given for not using mental health services, while lack of faith in the efficacy of mental health services was the least cited reason.

Clearly, researchers, policy makers, and providers emphasize the need to reduce and eliminate mental health disparities. Programmatic efforts are underway to bring to scale successful interventions that increase quality and access to mental health care for diverse populations, with focus on individual-, community-, provider-, and health system–related mechanisms underlying disparities in mental health status and psychiatric service use. Culturally adapted interventions using care managers, improved treatment initiation, patient activation, and self-management among minorities with limited English proficiency and limited health literacy are strategies used to decrease disparities (NIMHD, 2015). Also, community-partnered participatory research (CPPR) using a collaborative care model—which consisted of team approaches that use case managers to link primary care providers, patients, and mental health specialists—has shown improved mental health quality of life and reduced hospitalizations for mental disorders for all groups.

Some research indicates that racial and ethnic minority clients/patients may prefer same race and ethnic psychotherapists. Constantine (2001) investigated multicultural competence by having participants (clients) evaluate therapists using audiotaped sessions. Participants completed competence scales that evaluated the clinicians' multicultural counseling awareness, multicultural counseling knowledge, multicultural counseling skills, sociopolitical awareness, and cultural sensitivity. Results showed that clients rated African American and Latinx American counselors as significantly more multiculturally competent compared with European American therapists.

Knowledge About Pervasive Microaggressions and Privilege

Awareness and knowledge are important in mediating the propensity of individuals to commit microaggressions and to interact in covertly discriminatory ways, including in the psychotherapeutic intervention process. We all sometimes engage in hurtful behaviors because it has not occurred to us those certain behaviors are hurtful. Derald Wing Sue and his students have a body of research that examines the experience of microaggressions (Sue et al., 2019). *Microaggression* is a term used to describe power dynamics in cross-cultural interactions that express attitudes of dominance, superiority, and denigration, that a person with privilege is better than the person of color, who "is less than" (Fouad & Arredondo, 2007; D. W. Sue, 2003). Microaggressions are frequently committed by well-intentioned people who hold egalitarian values but who are not aware of the pejorative attitudes and stereotypes they hold about people of color and/or who have had insufficient interactions with people who are culturally different from them (Fouad & Arredondo, 2007). Strategies to "disarm" microaggressions are part of important skill sets for psychotherapists as well as for clients, and training in these strategies is valuable toward that endeavor (D. W. Sue et al., 2019).

Environmental microaggressions occur when a subtle discrimination occurs within society. An example would be a college campus that has multiple statues of Confederate heroes or a psychotherapy office that is experienced as invalidating if it is perceived as cold and unwelcoming. A psychotherapist who is a sports fan may be oblivious to the offensiveness of having Native caricatures as sports symbols in their office. We must realize that when clients feel empathy within the therapeutic environment, significant positive change outcome is more likely (Bohart et al., 2002).

Destructive processes such as microaggressions are unconscious at times, until we work to make them conscious. Multicultural competence is partly about the commitment to develop compassion for those different from us; it is a humanity inherent in the discipline of psychology. This requires that we talk more about what therapeutic effectiveness involves.

All of us engage in microaggressions. For example, Dr. V was a perpetrator during a meeting of former American Psychological Association (APA) president Ron Levant's Task Force on Enhancing Diversity. One of the main charges to this task force was to increase APA's "welcomeness" to diverse groups. One of our task force members uses a wheelchair for mobility, and on the first of two evenings, we made sure to go to a restaurant that was accessible. Even though it was accessible, the access for people in wheelchairs was around the back and through the kitchen because the front entrance had six steps. We did not notice that until our colleague, Rhoda Olkin (who gave me permission to use her name and to share this story), who was using her crutches that night, pointed it out. On the second night, she chose to rest and not attend our dinner. It was unspoken, but we went to a restaurant that was not accessible; in fact, we had chosen it and rejected it the night before to accommodate Rhoda. The next day, when Rhoda realized that we attended a restaurant that wasn't accessible, it was clear to me when I observed her reactions that our doing so was hurtful. Later in the day, she recommended that we encourage APA to not hold meetings in hotels, buildings, or restaurants that were not accessible *whether a person with disabilities was present or not*, just as we would not hold meetings at any place that barred women, Latinx, or religious groups. The community with disabilities would want our support to avoid inaccessible structures not only to make a statement but also to advocate for change. Here was a gathering of psychologists, handpicked because of our expertise and sensitivity to diversity, and we were all insensitive to this issue.

These insensitive microaggressions and processes are unconscious at times until someone points them out, and we work to make them conscious. Some people may resent the responsibility implied in this story, that is, to require accommodations when no one is directly affected, but this is indeed what commitment to diversity is about, as well as the commitment to compassion for humanity inherent in the discipline of psychology. A true ally "walks the talk" when no one is monitoring.

Knowledge of the Impact of Stress From
Poverty and Discrimination

Researchers have contributed to increasing our understanding of the impact of early life stress on the developing brain at the molecular and circuit levels across the life course among racially diverse groups (NIMHD, 2015). For example, the neuroscience of poverty was reported in the proceedings of the National Academy of Sciences (Katsnelson, 2015). While social science researchers have revealed a predictive link between children's socioeconomic status and lifelong health outcomes, academic achievement, and mental health, many questions remain. For example, if growing up in poverty has a negative impact on brain development in childhood, is it reversible? What are the specific underlying causes (Katsnelson, 2015)? Clarity is important because of important policy implications, such as social programs, that can alter the paths of poor families for the better.

The Adverse Childhood Experiences (ACE) Study (Felitti et al., 1998), conducted by the U.S. health maintenance organization Kaiser Permanente and the CDC, took a long-term look at health outcomes. It, along with numerous other studies (Barile et al., 2014; Metzler et al., 2017; Sheats et al., 2018), found a relationship between adverse childhood experiences (e.g., chronic physical and emotional abuse and neglect, sexual abuse, domestic violence, an incarcerated family member, substance use in household) with health and social problems across the lifespan. The ACE study has produced more than 50 publications that look at the prevalence and consequences of ACEs. Further, there is an intergenerational link. Merrick and Guinn (2018) reported that people who experience childhood adversity are more likely than those who do not to have children who have similar childhood experiences. Poverty begets poverty, violence begets violence, and so on.

Neuroscience has provided new potential explanations for the effects of poverty. The hippocampus, a key structure for consolidating memories, is loaded with stress hormone receptors. Apparently, socioeconomic status does not affect cognition across the board, but deficits are found to cluster in functions thought to engage specific brain circuits, including language, certain dimensions of memory, and the ability to regulate thoughts and emotions. However, understanding the developmental sequelae of poverty and whether or how children's developing brains compensate for it will necessitate complex studies that account for specific individual differences in children's responses to poverty (Blair & Raver, 2016).

Knowledge About Racial Profiling: Still Two Americas

Black and White Americans differ widely in their views of the criminal justice system, possibly because of such different and disparate experiences in their respective communities; one could say we have two different Americas. A Pew Research Center survey (Gramlich, 2019) found that Black Americans are far more likely than Whites to say that the criminal justice system is racially biased and that its treatment of minorities is a serious national problem.

Social psychologist Jennifer Eberhardt has conducted a series of experiments using brain imaging technology to show how mostly unconscious racial stereotypes can criminalize African Americans (Eberhardt, 2005). Using images of faces and objects flashed across a screen at speeds that range from subliminal to perceptible, Eberhardt discovered that subliminal exposure to a Black face led participants to better detect blurry images of weapons, while on the other hand, a White face inhibited detection of those objects.

Eberhardt's (2005) research also found that the "Blacker" a defendant appears—as measured by skin pigmentation, hair texture, and lip size—the more likely it was that the defendant would receive the death penalty than if the defendant were White. She also found that police officers are more likely to criminalize those people whose faces are the most stereotypically Black. According to Eberhardt, it is almost as if people are thinking of Blackness as a crime. Eberhardt and others are working with law enforcement agencies to improve policing and to counter implicit bias.

Even when human judgment is replaced by computer models, for example, criminal justice algorithms used to inform decisions on pretrial release and paroling, Lum and Johndrow (2016) found that "race-neutral models" still resulted in racially disparate predictions. Garcia (2016), who writes on biased and inappropriate utilization of data, reported that companies and government institutions that use data need to pay attention to the unconscious and institutional biases that seep into their results. She noted that with the proliferation of artificial intelligence, humans risk inserting their own biases into codes that will automatically make decisions for years to come. While end users of these codes may not hold the prejudices that produce distorted results in web searches, data-driven property loan decisions, or face-recognition software, it takes distorted inputs that the uninformed end user will not notice, and not make appropriate corrections to, that will result in biased outcomes.

Structural, institutional, and systemic racism refer to the system of procedures or processes that disadvantage Black, Indigenous, People of Color (BIPOC). These are both theoretical concepts as well as realities. The problems are complex, but the reality is that attention to and vigilance for pervasive biases are burdens that create an allostatic load for BIPOC. As psychologists and mental health providers, we have a responsibility to have knowledge about these realities for the populations with whom we work.

Knowledge About Institutional Violence Toward Mexicans and Mexican Americans

Although the history of slavery and its horrific aftermath is known to most readers, less well known is the historical and contemporary institutional violence toward Mexicans and Mexican Americans in this country. According to an article by Richard Delgado (2009), "Law of the Noose: A History of Latino Lynching," there are believed to have been roughly 600 lynchings of Mexicans and Mexican Americans beginning with the aftermath of the 1848 Treaty of Guadalupe-Hidalgo (the document that ended the Mexican American war, where Mexico ceded half of its land to the United States) between the years 1846 and 1925 throughout the Southwest United States. In this regard, the history of Blacks and Mexicans in the United States was similar as both groups were lynched by Anglos for the specious accusations of "acting uppity," taking jobs away from Anglos, provocatively eying Anglo women, cheating at cards, practicing "witchcraft," and refusing to leave homestead lands that Whites coveted. Furthermore, Mexicans were lynched for acting "too Mexican," for speaking Spanish, or for proudly celebrating aspects of their culture. Some Mexican women were lynched for resisting the sexual assaults of Anglo men. Law enforcement, especially the Texas Rangers, who had particular hatred toward individuals of Mexican descent, actively participated in many of these lynchings.

Mass deportations of immigrant children and adults, separation of children from their families at the border and forcing American citizen children into foster care without ways to track their location, and the refusal to allow asylum seekers into the country resulting in border camps are contemporary examples of violent and discriminatory policies that have negative impacts on the lives of immigrants and the communities in which they and their families live (Soboroff, 2020).

Efforts to make English the official language of the United States and to end bilingual education, thereby requiring immigrants to assimilate to the majority Anglo culture, have postcolonial scholars contending that movements to extinguish native languages facilitate children's acquisition of English as their dominant language and rejection of their cultural heritages. Delgado (2009) warned that these actions are an implicit form of lynching that have negative consequences to the individual and communities. This history is important to know as it continues to have an impact.

Knowledge About the Imposter Syndrome/Phenomenon

The *imposter syndrome* or imposter phenomenon is an ongoing fear, often experienced by high-achieving individuals, that they are going to be "found out" or unmasked as being incompetent or unable to replicate past successes (Abramson, 2021). Although up to 82% of the population faces those kinds of feelings, Black, Asian, Native American, and Latinx college students may particularly experience them, according to Cokley et al. (2017), who further described how BIPOC who work or study in predominantly White environments are especially vulnerable to struggling with imposter feelings. Imposter feelings are strongly linked to increased anxiety and depression. Those feelings can be conquered through individual efforts (share feelings with safe allies, develop support networks, celebrate successes, let go of perfectionism, cultivate self-compassion, share failures and realize they are a part of life), but they can also be minimized in how systems and settings promote the environmental culture. For example, a school or work setting can foster collaboration and support rather than toxic competitiveness. Authority figures in all walks of life, from educational institutions to industry and government, must consider how their official and unofficial policies and procedures disengage and "other" underrepresented people, preventing access, opportunity, and engagement in their systems.

MULTICULTURAL SKILLS

Various therapeutic skills are especially important in multicultural therapy. Empathy, which may be more challenging with those clients different from us, is especially important. Empathy is influenced by awareness and knowledge as discussed in previous sections but is essentially an important therapeutic skill. The ability to support and facilitate clients when they experience and perceive bias and stereotype threat are also critical skills. One of the most destructive interventions would be to try to convince the client that perpetrators did not really mean the offense, microaggression, etc. These skills are further discussed next.

Development of Empathy

While researchers have found that people experience a decreased sense of empathy for someone who is experiencing distress due to an incident arising from unfamiliar cultural norms, perspective taking on the part of the observer mediates this reduction in empathy (Batson et al., 2002; Bruneau & Saxe, 2012; Nelson & Baumgarte, 2004). These findings suggest that prior experiences and lack of similarity between two people can have a negative impact on the ability to understand and empathize from someone else's perspective (Opotow, 1990; Weng et al., 2013), and they also imply that exposure to and increasing familiarity with diverse cultures can improve empathy. Weng et al. (2013) found that compassion can be cultivated through training and that greater altruistic behavior may emerge from increased engagement of neural systems associated with the suffering of other people, executive and emotional control, and reward processing.

Missed empathetic opportunities in therapeutic encounters may be more frequent when clinicians and their clients have different cultural identities (Comas-Díaz, 2006). A good suggestion is to learn the client's uses of words to facilitate and guide learning of a new common language, as well as to teach the client concepts in the therapeutic dialogue. When we "stretch" our empathic skills on a regular basis, especially when we are experiencing negative judgment, even if someone or some situation is problematic, understanding their worldview and conveying that understanding before challenging them is worthwhile.

Walker (2020) described awareness, respect, and compassion as three transformative processes that aid in the promotion of empathy and enlarge our capacity to cultivate more authentic relationships with one another. Awareness conveys to the client that they have been heard. Respect takes us beyond sympathy or sentimentality and conveys an invitation to share more. Despite possible differences, respect creates conditions for growth. Compassion is an intentional acknowledgment of shared humanity and the antidote to contempt. Walker described these processes as the "ARC of empathy" (p. 68). These processes can help traverse an otherwise empathy deficit when the capacity to convey empathy is threatened by different, difficult encounters.

Cultural Humility

Cultural humility is described as different from cultural competency and as involving the ability to be flexible and humble enough to assess anew the cultural dimensions of the experiences of each patient (Tervalon & Murray-García, 1998). *Humility* is the freedom from pride or arrogance and can be defined as an ongoing process of self-reflection and self-critique to build honest and trustworthy relationships (Yeager & Bauer-Wu, 2013). It is a process whereby individuals not only learn about another's culture but also examine their own beliefs and cultural identities. Awareness of and sensitivity to historic realities, including histories resulting in mistrust such as those described previously in this chapter, contribute to the practice of cultural humility (Sufrin, 2019).

Perceiving and Reducing Bias, Stereotype Threat, and Microaggressions

Living in a society that devalues one's identity group can have many unintended consequences. Steele's (1997, 2011) "stereotype threat" research indicated that when ethnic minorities are asked to perform a task in which ethnic minorities stereotypically are perceived to underperform, regardless of their actual ability to perform, they ultimately underperform *because* of the threat/fear/anxiety of underperforming. Ethnic minority clients may experience negative judgment, rejection, and criticalness on the part of White therapists without the White therapists being aware of this. Therapists must take special precautions not to "prejudge" the client by conflating problems with ethnicity. Because of a history of oppressive and rejecting experiences, many ethnic minorities are vulnerable to feeling shamed, and an unaware psychotherapist may not know when they unconsciously communicate negative judgments through their body language (Greenwald & Banaji, 1995).

It is critical that individuals be supported to respond with healthy coping skills to those normal but painful life events that everyone unfortunately experiences. The use of cognitive techniques, such as reframing and perspective taking, can help a client through this process. Therapist-selected self-disclosure of similar experiences of failures or mistakes and our reactions to them may help normalize these moments in our lives and assure that we survive painful mistakes, failures, or rejections.

D. W. Sue et al.'s (2019) microintervention strategies can help clients learn to disarm and dismantle microaggressions. A therapist could first help a client recognize microaggressions; many times, individuals feel hurt or ashamed or embarrassed in an interaction and may not even recognize when and how the offense has occurred: "I bet you got your promotion because of affirmative action." D. W. Sue et al. (2019) identified four major goals of microinterventions: (a) make the invisible visible, (b) disarm the microaggression, (c) educate the perpetrator, and (d) seek external rein-forcement or support. Role playing or practicing the microinterventions can be helpful. Additionally, the therapist can support and apply those skills in the context of therapy with the therapist as well!

SUMMARY

This chapter has suggested that the theory of multicultural therapy involves the description of how competence is developed within the context of three overarching domains that define the multiculturally competent psycho-therapist: awareness, knowledge, and skills. They are thus goals in the ongoing quest to gain and maintain the competence that includes under-standing the influence of cultures, contexts, and systemic issues on clients and therapists as well as on the process and outcome of therapy. We realize that the process of developing multicultural therapy competence is a complex, developmental, and ongoing process that involves not only a way of doing therapy with multicultural clients but also a way of being with clients in psychotherapy. More strategies and skills are described in the next chapter, which focuses on the process of multicultural therapy.

4

Therapeutic Process: Primary Change Mechanisms

Attention to the change process and the relative significance of culturally specific versus universal approaches to psychotherapy are important to discuss. Fischer et al. (1998) addressed the tension that exists in the literature between emic (culturally specific) and etic (universal) approaches to counseling with culturally different clients. They suggested that both were important and relevant and described universal healing conditions, those in the common factors approach to treatment in culturally specific contexts. In other words, the common factors found in conventional psychotherapy and in healing across cultures, combined with a thorough knowledge of cultural context, can effectively be considered competent multicultural counseling. The American Psychological Association's definition of evidence-based practice in psychology calls for consideration of both: "Evidence based practice in psychology is the integration of the best available research with clinical expertise in the context

https://doi.org/10.1037/0000279-004
Multicultural Therapy: A Practice Imperative, by M. J. T. Vasquez and J. D. Johnson
Copyright © 2022 by the American Psychological Association. All rights reserved.

of patient characteristics, culture and preferences" (APA Presidential Task Force on Evidence-Based Practice, 2006, p. 273). It is possible that more acculturated clients would respond well to the etic approaches, and clients with lower acculturation levels would respond better to the emic approaches, those with cultural adaptations.

Frank and Frank (1991) identified four "common factors" as critical to psychotherapeutic effectiveness: the therapeutic relationship; a shared worldview (here defined as beliefs and attitudes about life and the world that inform thoughts and behaviors); client expectations; and the "ritual," or interventions, of the psychotherapeutic process itself. Wampold (2015) suggested that a contextual model for psychotherapy is important to understanding the evidence that these common factors are salient for producing the benefits of psychotherapy. He identified common factors within a contextual model to include the (a) real relationship; (b) creation of expectations through an explanation of the client's problems, how they developed, and how they may be resolved; and (c) enactment of health promoting actions. Wampold (2015) also described the importance of the common factors that researchers using meta-analytic methodologies have identified as critical to psychotherapeutic effectiveness: the alliance, empathy, expectations, cultural adaptations, and therapist differences.

This chapter addresses the therapeutic process and primary change mechanisms by highlighting the role of the therapist–client relationship, the role of the therapist, and the role of the client. The models of therapeutic change such as the common factors inform our discussions. We provide a longer case study to try to demonstrate those change mechanisms. In doing so, we illustrate how the multicultural therapeutic process occurs, resulting in effective change for clients.

ROLE OF THE THERAPIST–CLIENT RELATIONSHIP

The most important of the common factors has been identified as the therapeutic relationship, or therapeutic alliance. This vital element is present across all psychotherapies and healing relationships in all cultures. Frank and Frank (1991) described it as "an emotionally charged, confiding relationship with a helping person" (p. 40). A trusting relationship between client and psychotherapist is a basic necessity in providing hope and improvement in counseling; the personal qualities of the therapist such as warmth, genuineness, and empathy work to enhance the quality of this relationship (Fischer et al., 1998). Cultural awareness and knowledge of the client's cultural context are needed to facilitate this trust and connection to accurately convey the warmth, genuineness, and empathy in a manner that is meaningful to the client.

As discussed previously, empathy is a critical factor and plays a central role in psychotherapy effectiveness. In previous chapters, we discussed how awareness of one's attitude and way of being with the client, influenced by attention to the cultural context, converges to create a complex, dynamic construct (S. B. Gibbons, 2011). The quality of empathic engagement between the psychotherapist and client is grounded in a shared, embodied humanity (S. B. Gibbons, 2011). In a meta-analytic study, Bohart et al. (2002) demonstrated the relationship between empathy and psychotherapy outcome, finding that psychotherapist empathy is key to the change process in therapy. Understanding a client's culture at the deeper levels can help promote this empathy within the therapist (Ani, 1994; Pope et al., 2021).

Multiculturally trained psychotherapists who understand the unique cultures and values of their clients sometimes cross boundaries in psychotherapy. In the therapist–client relationship, it is helpful to distinguish between the concepts of boundary crossings and boundary violations. Attitudes and behaviors that detract from therapists' objectivity in their work with their clients may represent a boundary crossing. These attitudes and behaviors may be helpful or harmful. For example, a therapist makes an exception to their ordinary practice and visits their client's home for a session. Does it make a difference if the therapist is sexually attracted to that client versus if that client is in hospice? It does. A boundary violation is one that is harmful to the therapeutic relationship by exploiting or violating the safety of the client. The notion of boundaries has evolved as an important strategy of "doing no harm" because the needs of the psychologist could potentially obstruct therapy. It is the therapist's responsibility to know which behaviors harm and which behaviors help the client and the therapeutic alliance.

While the APA (2017a) *Ethical Principles of Psychologists and Code of Conduct* (Standard 3.05, Multiple Relationships) describes harm that can result from boundary violations, the relevant standard also suggests that not all boundary crossings are unethical. The evolution of this standard was partly the result of members who argued that cultural values sometimes allowed for crossing boundaries such as those described below. Standard 3.05 states:

> (a) A multiple relationship occurs when a psychologist is in a professional role with a person and (1) at the same time is in another role with the same person, (2) at the same time is in a relationship with a person closely associated with or related to the person with whom the psychologist has the professional relationship, or (3) promises to enter into another relationship in the future with the person or a person closely associated with or related to the person.
>
> A psychologist refrains from entering into a multiple relationship if the multiple relationship could reasonably be expected to impair the psychologist's objectivity, competence, or effectiveness in performing his or her functions as a psychologist, or otherwise risks exploitation or harm to the person with whom the professional relationship exists.
>
> Multiple relationships that would not reasonably be expected to cause impairment or risk exploitation or harm are not unethical.
>
> (b) If a psychologist finds that, due to unforeseen factors, a potentially harmful multiple relationship has arisen, the psychologist takes reasonable steps to resolve it with due regard for the best interests of the affected person and maximal compliance with the Ethics Code. (p. 6)

Part of being culturally competent means knowing how to appropriately engage around common interactions, such as gift exchanges, attending clients' life events, responding to inquiries requiring self-disclosure, and nonsexual touch. Can maintaining strict boundaries contribute to increasing the risk of harm? We believe so. A Latinx psychotherapist, comfortable with hugging other Latinx members of the community, would not reject a client who stepped forward to hug their therapist at the end of a powerful session. Multicultural ethicists interpret boundary maintenance in the therapeutic relationship on a continuum rather than binary (Corey &

Herlihy, 2015). Exceptions to established professional boundaries must be compatible with one's theoretical conceptualization and informed by multicultural therapy theory and the cultural contexts in which one is working. We encourage consultation with knowledgeable colleagues as well as articulation of the exception documented in treatment process notes (Barnett et al., 2007).

ROLE OF THE PSYCHOTHERAPIST

One of the most important roles of the psychotherapist is to promote the four common factors identified by Frank and Frank (1991) and described previously in this chapter, including the establishment of the bond, connection, and alliance involved in the therapeutic relationship; a shared worldview (the client experiences your understanding of theirs); client expectations (they trust that you "get" and understand their problems, what caused them, and what can help); and the "ritual," or interventions, of the psychotherapeutic process itself. We believe that the process of promoting those four factors requires that the psychotherapist acquire, develop, and apply their own multicultural awareness, knowledge, and skills in working with each individual client.

Reduction of Bias

A multicultural therapist is committed to the ongoing reduction of bias within themselves, their colleagues, and their clients. One develops an antiracist identity by first acknowledging that one's racist beliefs exists; this requires the tolerance of the unpleasant experience of engaging in an honest appraisal of one's biases and prejudices (D. W. Sue, 2003). When we deny our own racism, we make it more difficult to understand our racial and cultural selves, and we cannot therefore develop an integrated authentic identity. In addition, we must not continue to view racial and ethnic minority individuals and groups as "disloyal aliens in their own country" (D. W. Sue, 2003, p. xiii). Frequently, especially during stressful times, people blame and scapegoat others. We previously discussed how, during the COVID-19 crisis in 2020, several members of the Asian

American community were attacked and victimized verbally and physically based on the belief that the virus originated in China, and that they were somehow at fault. Another example was the scapegoating of Middle Eastern communities after the assault on the United States on September 11, 2001. This scapegoating phenomenon is prevalent when we categorize people based on stereotypes, blame victims for their plight, and maintain an outgroup bias of negatively treating those who are perceived as different (Chin, 2020). Finally, multicultural experts recommend that every individual, not just people of color, is responsible for combating racism in ourselves and in society at large (D. W. Sue, 2003).

Antiracism

Most people do not want to be considered racist or biased in any way, but they spend more of their time seeking to avoid those labels rather than exploring their attitudes, beliefs, and behavior and the ways that they have been advantaged by systems of interrelated privilege and oppression (Green, 2007). Although we are not personally responsible for the existence of these systems of privilege and disadvantage, we do move within them all the time (Green, 2007); thus, we are all responsible for acknowledging the presence of social privileges in our lives and the ways we benefit from them. Failure to acknowledge opportunities and privilege, or the lack of those, is evident when we hear people blame unemployed individuals for not securing work, for example. The complexities of dealing with insidious bias and institutional racism are often critical factors in understanding who has access to opportunities and who does not. This was nicely captured in an old bumper sticker that read, "Racism: Our National Disease. Getting sick was not our fault. Getting well is our responsibility."

How do we take responsibility for our antiracism and racial equity change processes? Let us begin by looking at the science. Results from a classic large meta-analysis indicate that higher levels of intergroup contact are associated with lower levels of intergroup prejudice, and these effects are stronger when optimal conditions are established within the contact situation (e.g., equal status between groups, supportive institutional norms—laws, policies, etc.; Allport, 1954). We also know that positive contact effects emerge largely because the contact helps to reduce anxiety and increase empathy between groups, which in turn contributes to reduced prejudice (Pettigrew & Tropp, 2008). Another strategy is to change the perception of "us versus them" to "we," or recategorizing the outgroup as members of the ingroup (Gaertner & Dovidio, 2000). This was found to be effective, particularly under conditions of low bias and where interpersonal communication was the focus (Hewstone et al., 2002).

We all have clients whom we respect, as well as clients whom we do not, perhaps unconsciously. Sometimes these feelings are based on client personality variables or their attitudes, beliefs, and behaviors, all of which are grist for the therapeutic mill. Other times, our failure to feel respect for our clients may be a result of our biases, which a client may never be able to overcome. To change this, an important constructive strategy is to assume the individual is worthy of being perceived as in our ingroup. Our therapeutic stance of tuning into our clients, listening to their stories, and connecting with them empathically can help us overcome our biases by suspending and managing our pejorative assessments and negative reactions.

Personal Qualities of Effective Therapists

Ackerman and Hilsenroth (2003) and Norcross and Lambert (2011) identified therapists' personal characteristics and in-session behaviors that positively influenced the therapeutic alliance from a wide variety of psychotherapeutic orientations. Personal qualities found to make a positive contribution to the alliance include being adaptable, honest, respectful, trustworthy, confident, warm, curious, and open. These authors also identified specific therapeutic strategies that contribute to a positive alliance, including exploration, creating opportunities for contemplation, noting therapeutic progress, accurate interpretation, facilitating the expression of affect, and attending to the patient's experiences. Furthermore, effective therapists are able to form stronger alliances across a range of clients, have a greater level of facilitative interpersonal skills, express more professional self-doubt (expression of humility, perhaps?), and engage in more time outside of the actual therapy honing various therapy skills (Wampold, 2015).

Although these attributes and techniques may work with clients who are Black, Indigenous, People of Color (BIPOC), Comas-Díaz (2006) suggested careful application of any evidence-based findings in psychotherapy in general since there is a paucity of this type of research with populations of color. Furthermore, we don't know if ethnic and racial minorities from the general population respond similarly to different therapeutic approaches and interventions as do the individuals typically used in analogue research (e.g., undergraduates). For example, some ethnic and racial minority clients may find the horizontal relationship and nondirective interaction styles of some therapists confusing. Because of the dearth of evidence-based or empirically validated treatments on ethnic and racial minorities, careful attention must be paid to the nuances that education, socioeconomic status, acculturation, language, generational status, and other factors (APA, 2003) play in the experiences of bias and expressions of distress that may result. What we can assume is that our delivery of psychotherapeutic services needs to be responsive to the psychological sequelae that results from these experiences. For example, therapists using cognitive behavioral approaches may need to assess the role of racism and oppression in their client's ability to achieve mastery and agency. Teaching racial stress management strategies may be empowering coping skills for BIPOC clients who experience discrimination and microaggressions.

Multicultural Orientation: Way of Being, Cultural Humility

Owen (2013) introduced the concept of *multicultural orientation* (MCO) to include cultural humility, opportunities and missed opportunities, and cultural comfort. He suggested that the tripart model of multicultural competencies of knowledge, skills, and awareness should be foundational in treatment, but that the expression of those varies. MCO is described as a "way of being" with the client, while multicultural competencies describe a "way of doing." MCO describes how well a therapist engages in and implements multicultural awareness and knowledge. Cultural humility is an other-oriented perspective that involves respect, lack of superiority, and attunement. Cultural opportunities are those that allow a therapist to explore a client's cultural heritage, often overlooked, avoided, and invalidated within mainstream institutions and systems. Cultural comfort leads to increased probability of the elicitation and exploration of the client's cultural identity and experiences. Owen acknowledged that these constructs overlap with the concepts of the development of the alliance, and with the notion of empathy, but articulating, understanding, and incorporating the distinct construct of MCO is useful for our focus.

We are aware that as psychotherapists who are BIPOC, many of our clients who are BIPOC choose to come to see us because of our race and ethnic identities. Other BIPOC, with internalized racism, might choose to avoid seeing someone like us. Internalized racism involves both conscious and unconscious acceptance of a racial hierarchy in which White people are consistently ranked above people of color (Johnson, 2008). Thus, these clients may prefer a White psychotherapist, with the conscious or unconscious belief that a BIPOC would not be as competent as a White counselor.

We are also aware that many of our White American clients have to go through a process of resolving their cognitive dissonance to assume our competency, because if they grew up in this society, people from our race and ethnic backgrounds are largely not assumed to be competent. What happens when we, as women of BIPOC identities, have clients who are angry at affirmative action policies or at the Black Lives Matter movement, and make derogatory statements about racial and ethnic minorities, or perhaps even about members of our identity groups, such as race and ethnicity or gender?

How do we resolve this dissonance? Dr. J had an occasion to participate in an APA Annual Convention workshop addressing the question "What were you thinking?" She interviewed a number of her White clients to ascertain why they knowingly chose a female therapist of color. They gave a variety of responses, including the strength of the referral recommendation, the presumption of competency given her credentials, even the sound of her voice on the office voicemail message. A number of them insisted that race and ethnicity were never factors. Taking competency as a given, some were reassured by the belief that there was less likelihood of encountering the therapist in their social circles.

A basic responsibility for ethical practice is to keep in mind the human dignity of those with whom we work (Pope & Vasquez, 1998). Therefore, our primary task with the client whose anger is expressed through racist comments is to attend to the client's pain, anxiety, and fears in the context of the client's experience. It may be that at some point, later in the moment, session, or course of therapy, issues regarding transference and countertransference and/or addressing the impact of the client's insensitive methods of dealing with pain can be processed. But the primary responsibility is to attend to the client's core issues and to later address the client's biases and how we perceive and experience them. Green (2007) suggested that monitoring our humanity involves being mindful of someone else's susceptibility to injury or harm stemming from our actions and vice versa. We must pay extra close attention when the power dynamics in the therapy room shift in our favor as we must not let our client's -isms influence our professional judgment and intervention. Each therapist must determine when a client's racism is too vitriolic or destructive to one's health and welfare. In such a situation, because our clinical objectivity may become compromised, referring the client to another professional may be in everyone's best interests.

In a dynamic analysis, Comas-Díaz and Jacobsen (1995) discussed the interracial dyad involving a therapist of color and a White patient, exploring the issues of power and transferential and countertransferential reactions. They suggested this dyad provides an opportunity for ethnic and racial minority therapists to understand the perspectives, realities, and experiences of their White patients and, by extension, White people in general. Similarly, our White clients can benefit from understanding the worldviews, experiences of unearned disadvantages, and intersectionalities of their therapists of color. Both members of the dyad can learn from and appreciate each other.

An older White man telephoned Dr. V inquiring about the opportunity of exploring the possibility of engaging her services. The potential client inquired extensively about her background, training, years of experience, and approach to treatment. He reported that he had both medical and law degrees. The therapist's automatic reaction was to address her own anxiety by pathologizing and labeling him as paranoid and obsessive-compulsive. After a few moments, the therapist was able to engage in a healthier, and likely more accurate, assessment that included compassionately acknowledging that this was his first attempt at psychotherapy, and that he was uncomfortable being vulnerable and asking for help. The *APA Guidelines for Psychological Practice With Boys and Men* (2018a) remind us that adherence to traditional masculinity is associated with reluctance to seek psychological help. Both the psychotherapist's reaction and reframe are grist for the psychotherapeutic mill and can benefit the psychotherapist and client.

The *Multicultural Guidelines* (APA, 2003, 2017b) ask us to acknowledge differences and, even if they make us uncomfortable, be respectful about them. We have all had experiences in which our critical, negative judgments and perceptions were misplaced, inappropriate, and unfounded, and we must be cautious as to whether such stances are ever legitimate in the psychotherapy room. If not, the ethical mandate is to refer (APA, 2017a, Standard 2.01b, Boundaries of Competence).

ROLE OF THE CLIENT

The third common factor in the behavior change process involves the role of the client, including the client expectations. Clients often come to psychotherapy demoralized and distressed and have often attempted to cope with their problems unsuccessfully. They thus come to psychotherapy hopeful that they will be given solutions. Effective multicultural therapy helps provide the client with an explanation and elucidation of ways to cope with and overcome their difficulties. The better the psychotherapist–client bond and relationship, the more similar the worldview, and the more the client will trust and believe that the psychotherapy process will be helpful. The client's positive expectations that counseling will relieve their distress or problems enhance the probability of success. When a psychotherapist provides the client with a plausible explanation for their distress, the client's positive hopes and expectations about therapy will likely increase (Fischer et al., 1998). Clients who are able to develop constructive expectations and believe their psychotherapist to be credible are more likely to have positive outcomes. The psychotherapist supports the client through the context of the therapeutic environment, their credentials and professionalism, working within the client's worldview, and developing an efficacious therapeutic alliance (Fischer et al., 1998; Wampold, 2015).

BRIEF AND LONG-TERM STRATEGIES AND TECHNIQUES

The fourth common factor, interventions or rituals, follows from the previous three factors of the roles of the therapeutic relationship, a shared worldview, and client expectations. Frank and Frank (1991) proposed that there are an infinite number of rituals, strategies, techniques, and interventions that can be used with a client, so long as those chosen are efficacious, believable, and culturally relevant to the client. We describe those interventions we believe to be especially important for multicultural psychotherapists.

Identify Areas of Strength and Resilience

When people are in pain, they sometimes forget to put things in perspective, focusing solely on the cause of their distress. Each of us has a fundamental need to be reminded of our worth, particular strengths, and capacity for resilience. Fortunately, many psychotherapy orientations incorporate elements of positive psychology and strengths-based approaches in their therapeutic practices. Feminist and multicultural therapies further emphasize the identification and elimination of systemic and institutional biases (thereby reframing the source of a "problem" from an individual to an institution, for example) and encourage interpersonal empowerment while working toward enhanced quality of life for all people.

Resilience is broadly defined as one's capacity to successfully adjust and adapt to adversity (DeNisco, 2011; Manning, 2013). Future research will hopefully shed light on the resilience, strengths, and survivorship of ethnic groups, despite various challenges (D. L. Brown, 2008; Vasquez & de las Fuentes, 1999). We do know that a variety of cultural factors may provide powerful sources of emotional resilience, for example, despite enduring poverty-level income, many Latinx people exhibit values and behaviors that include a strong belief in marriage and family, a vigorous work ethic, and a desire for education (Hayes-Bautista, 1992).

Many Latinx people, but especially women, have a higher life expectancy rate than any other group in this country. According to the Centers for Disease Control and Prevention (CDC) of the National Center for Health Statistics (Arias, 2016), for the female population, life expectancy increased for Hispanic women (from 83.8 to 84), remained unchanged for Black women (78.1), and decreased for White women (81.2 to 81.1). For the male population, life expectancy increased slightly between 2013 and 2014 for Hispanic men (from 79.1 to 79.2) and for non-Hispanic Black men (from 71.8 to 72) but remained unchanged for non-Hispanic White men (76.5). The hypotheses for the higher life expectancy for Hispanics include that because extended families provide emotional support, Hispanics, especially women, are less likely to live alone, are more likely to be caregivers of older and younger members of their families, less likely to be smokers or drinkers of alcohol, may have a better diet, and their infant mortality rate is lower than that of other groups. More research is needed to identify specific factors that buffer the negative experiences of the Hispanic population and give rise to longer lives. This phenomenon is called the "Hispanic paradox" since despite poverty and discrimination, they tend live longer than White or Black Americans. Kristof (2020) suggested that the resilience is likely a result of the emphasis on faith, family, and community ties and that this social fabric, while not a perfect shield from challenges such as the COVID-19 pandemic, is nonetheless a lesson for the rest of us.

Bilingualism may also contribute to resilience. Seniors between the ages of 60 and 68 who had spoken two languages for most of their lives were faster at switching from one mental task to another compared with monolingual seniors (Gold et al., 2013). Lifelong bilingualism can retain the youthful cognitive control abilities in later years and may offset age-related declines in the neural efficiency for cognitive control processes. For example, bilingualism may help mitigate certain dementias, such as Alzheimer's disease. These findings are comparable to those by Schachter et al. (2012), who found that across ethnic immigrants, being bilingual was associated with better physical and mental health relative to being proficient in only English or one's native language. The associations were mediated by socioeconomic status and family support but not by acculturation, stress and discrimination, or health access and behaviors.

Familismo, a Latino cultural value emphasizing strong family relationships, may be a buffer against depression by promoting positive social support even when faced with substantial environmental risk. Findings by Plant and Sachs-Ericsson (2004) may support this. In their meta-analysis on depression and racial and ethnic minorities, they found that interpersonal functioning served as a protective factor against depressive symptoms to a greater extent for Latinos and other minorities than for non-Latino White individuals. The phenomenon of the Hispanic/Latinx Paradox (Palloni & Morenoff, 2001) describes the unique resilience to the usual negative health outcomes resulting from poverty and related public health challenges, such as infant mortality and low birth weight, when contrasted with non-Latino White people and other groups. Although specific protective factors that may enhance Latino mental health have not yet been identified, family networks and spirituality have been hypothesized. It is important to note that this resilience may decrease as individuals acculturate in the United States (Plant & Sachs-Ericsson, 2004). Acculturation is apparently bad for one's health, and the burdens of poverty and discrimination result in effects that are not always mediated by resilience.

African American communities, including through Black churches, are also hypothesized to provide resilience in regard to depression associated with low socioeconomic status, poverty, and discrimination. Spirituality and religion play an important role in the lives of many African Americans, and the activities associated with them may provide beneficial effects on health and be a significant resilience factor for people living with life difficulties (Choi & Hastings, 2019; Pargament & Cummings, 2010). Resilient individuals have been found to have had better diabetes control, higher levels of positivity, and lower levels of depression (Steinhardt et al., 2015). More study is needed as the research is lacking, and the findings from one group cannot be generalized to another.

Although therapists are encouraged to be aware of barriers, obstacles, and experiences of oppression for our clients of color, it is also important to remain open to strengths, resilience, and positive aspects of identity. Listen for your clients' strengths and reflect those back regularly, as they may not see them in themselves.

Cultural Adaptations of Evidence-Based Practice

In the past 40 years, the proliferation of evidence-based and theoretical multicultural scholarship has strengthened the opportunities for mental health providers to adhere to the ethical requirements of developing their competencies in delivery of services to members of diverse groups. When you know more about culture, you are more able to engage in cultural adaptations of evidence-based practices. Bernal and Domenech Rodriguez (2012) described results from their meta-analysis of 65 experimental studies. They found that cultural adaptations of practice work better for people of color than traditional therapies; they reviewed many kinds of adaptations, including incorporating cultural content and values into treatment, using the client's preferred language, and matching clients with therapists of similar ethnicity and race.

Whaley and Davis (2007) suggested that the impact of culture may be most important during the development of the therapeutic alliance and that instrumental support and linguistic and content adaptations to the delivery of psychological services may be critical to the engagement and retention of the client in treatment. Miranda et al. (2006), for example, developed a culturally adapted treatment for low-income minority women with depression by providing child care and transportation. They also provided several psychoeducational sessions about depression and its treatment prior to delivering the culturally adapted cognitive behavior therapeutic interventions developed by Muñoz and Mendelson (2005). Whaley and Davis described the application of culturally relevant examples from Latino/a culture using *dichos* (or "sayings"), for example, the saying *la gota de agua labra la piedra* ("a drop of water carves a rock") to illustrate how even fleeting thoughts can influence one's view of life and cause and maintain depression. Cultural adaptation of evidence-based treatments may indeed make mental health services more culturally competent.

In his description of the contextual model of the common factors, Wampold (2015) concluded that adapting evidence-based treatments by using an explanation congruent with the client's cultural group's beliefs was more effective than unadapted evidence-based treatments. This fits the model that declares that explanations for the client's difficulties and distress as well as explanations about the strategies and solutions must be meaningful to the client.

Use of Interpreters

Unfortunately, using the client's preferred language may be challenging, as there are tremendous language diversities in the United States. The U.S. Census Bureau (2015) reported that while most of the U.S. population speaks only English at home or a handful of other languages such as Spanish or Vietnamese, at least 350 languages are spoken in U.S. homes, including 150 different North American Native and Indigenous languages, collectively spoken by more than 350,000 people. Furthermore, there is a gaping disparity between the percentage of linguistic minorities in the United States and the percentage of them prepared to deliver psychological health services (APA, 2016). For example, in 2016, there were about 57.5 million Hispanics in the United States, representing about 18% of the U.S. population. Forty million of these, or 72.4%, spoke Spanish in their homes (U.S. Census Bureau, 2017), yet only 5.5% of psychologists surveyed in that same year delivered services in Spanish (APA, 2016), exemplifying one of the biggest barriers to treatment for Spanish speakers.

Approximately 13% of the U.S. population are immigrants, many of whom seek psychological help. They face the stress of adaptation to a new culture, and some are asylum seekers or refugees dealing with the trauma of poverty, war, and natural disasters (DeAngelis, 2010). Faced with language differences, practitioners may rely on language interpreters to provide therapy. It is not considered a best practice to rely on family members, especially children, as interpreters. The use of interpreters can be a challenging option, and specific precautions should be considered when using them (Searight & Searight, 2009; Yakushko, 2010). Nonetheless, when bilingual therapists are not available, well-trained interpreters can make a significant difference in positive treatment outcomes, and training programs for mental health interpreters are available in various states (DeAngelis, 2010).

Quinn (2011) interviewed psychotherapists who had used interpreters. The psychotherapists described how the interpreter plays a major role in how clients from different cultures experience the psychotherapist and the psychotherapeutic process. Examples were provided where interpreters had a constructive or destructive impact on the work. Interpreters can form a natural dyad with the client due to shared language or culture; they can also affect the therapeutic relationship by adding or filtering meaning and misrepresenting the client or counselor to the other. A well-trained interpreter can help deepen understanding of the counseling process to the client and perhaps extend that understanding to the community.

Training interpreters for mental health work includes the provision of a basic understanding of the therapy process, the importance of understanding confidentiality and boundaries, and the importance of translating everything they hear, without filtering incoherence or discontinuity in speech, for example. Debriefing to discuss parts of the session that were confusing or difficult to translate can help provide insight into a client's condition (DeAngelis, 2010). The therapist's speaking in short phrases or words can be helpful to the interpreter. Building an alliance and bond with the interpreter can help facilitate the process, and maintaining the same interpreter throughout a psychotherapy relationship can facilitate a constructive experience for all.

The competent delivery of mental health services to language minority clients requires knowledge of their cultures and histories, culturally specific racial and ethnic identity development, variables that affect service delivery (e.g., immigration, citizenship status), and language fluency. Fortunately, there are now about a dozen psychology and counseling programs in the United States that train graduate students to deliver services to their language minority clients, specifically Spanish speakers (https://www.apa.org/monitor/2018/06/spanish-speaking-programs). The goals for these programs are to improve trainees' multicultural competencies and oral and written language proficiencies in psychology-related contexts (Biever et al., 2002, 2011).

The following case study illustrates a multicultural therapeutic change process, including a description of the relationship and the roles of the psychotherapist and the client in the process.[1]

LONGER CASE STUDY: CASE EXAMPLE OF CROSS-CULTURAL MULTICULTURAL THERAPY PROCESS WITH A BLACK MALE CLIENT

One of the authors, a Black female psychologist (Dr. J), had the opportunity to provide brief therapy to a patient, a Black male, referred by his regular therapist, a White female psychologist. Dr. J saw the patient, "Samuel," for brief supportive therapy while his regular therapist, Dr. R, was temporarily unavailable. Samuel returned to treatment with Dr. R and, 6 months later, Dr. J followed up with both to analyze and assess the impact of both therapeutic experiences. The unique circumstance provided an opportunity to explore some of the key issues in multicultural therapy: dynamics of race and gender differences in dyads; addressing spirituality; initiating discussions about race in the therapy session; dynamics of racial parity in therapeutic dyads; and cultural humility from multiple perspectives.

Using the ADDRESSING framework, a system of conceptualizing the multiple, complex, and contextual ways people identify themselves developed by P. A. Hays (2016), Samuel's identities are summarized in Table 4.1.

Samuel reported his educational status as "some college" but did not indicate a specific area of study. He said that he could never determine what he was interested in enough to pursue a four-year degree. He had some interest in police work but as that was the only area that was unacceptable to his mother, he did not pursue it.

---

[1] The confidentiality of the client has been maintained by changing significant identifiers; the dialogue is a composite construction used for instructional purposes.

Table 4.1

Samuel's Cultural Influences

Age and generational influences	66
Disability status (physical, cognitive, sensory, intellectual; acquired physical cognitive/ psychological disabilities)	No contributing health history
Diagnosis status	Initial: Unspecified Obsessive-Compulsive Disorder
	Working: Relational Distress With Spouse/ Intimate Partner
Religion and spiritual orientation	Nondenominational Christian faith
Ethnicity and race	Black
Socioeconomic status	Working class
Sexual orientation	Hetero-attractional
Indigenous heritage	None identified
National origin and current status	U.S. citizen; native born
Gender identity and expression	Cisgender male; masculine

Note. Adapted from *Addressing Cultural Complexities in Practice: Assessment, Diagnosis, and Therapy* (3rd ed., p. 8), by P. A. Hays, 2016, American Psychological Association (https://doi.org/10.1037/14801-000). Copyright 2016 by the American Psychological Association.

History

Samuel was the seventh of 10 children born in rural Tennessee. Both parents raised him. His father was employed primarily as a farm worker, and his mother was a homemaker. She was the primary disciplinarian who used the "switch" to mete out corporal punishment, although he did not recall it as being excessive. His father was 25 years older than his mother, a point that was to become meaningful later in Samuel's life. He did not endorse that his father was alcoholic, but like most of the men described in his community he went "out" to drink on the weekends. He described his father as having been busy in siring his 10 children from 1942 until 1960—the youngest child was born when the oldest was graduating high school. Samuel recalls that the "White" K–12 school in his town was made of red bricks while his school was made of cinderblocks. There were many other examples of resource inequities in his community.

Even though the family had limited resources, they "did not feel poor until TV showed them how poor they were." He added that TV today shows that no matter how much money the rich have, it's never enough. Samuel said, "I would rather be happy and poor than rich and unhappy." He noted that there was a lot of love in his house. Though he knows that they must have disagreed, Samuel does not recall ever hearing his parents argue. He says his mother was strong-willed and suspects that his father simply capitulated to her demands. This perhaps laid the foundation for the relational conflict he was to later describe.

At the age of 19, Samuel married his 18-year-old girlfriend. His mother's response when he told her of his plan has resonated with him his entire life. She did not challenge or criticize him for being too young. She showed her confidence in him by saying that it was his life, and he should do what he felt made him happy. His mother's worldview has shaped his own in significant ways. He still tries to live by the "golden rule" beliefs that she espoused even during Jim Crow days. She was never hypocritical; she was the same on weekdays as she was on Sunday. She demonstrated strength of character in quitting using "snuff" immediately upon hearing that it could cause cancer. Her willpower set a high exemplary standard for him. She shunned alcohol and never allowed it in her home. Recall that his father had to go "out" to drink with his friends on weekends. His mother died 3 years ago at the age of 90. His father died at age 67.

Samuel lived in Tennessee until he was 24 years old. He moved his family to Michigan and worked in the auto industry for 30 years. After retirement, he took his current position as a security officer. He has a good work ethic and attributes that in part to what he describes as his "OCD" (obsessive-compulsive disorder). He sees this as character strength, as it is important to "do things the right way."

Status

In 2014, Samuel's wife of 42 years died of cancer. He described their communication as "not good . . . we tended to sweep things under the rug." He has two grown daughters and two grandchildren. There has been a breakdown in his relationship with the youngest daughter who does not approve of his girlfriend. The relationship with said girlfriend was the focal point of his treatment with Dr. J. His connection to and involvement with his church rises above essentially everything else in his life.

Therapy

Samuel is a 66-year-old man who presented for treatment with Dr. R to address a history of addictive behaviors, grief and loss, relationship stress, and stage-of-life concerns related to loneliness. A friend recommended that Samuel seek out the self-help group Recovering Through Faith. It was there he met Dr. R, who was involved with the program. He approached her and asked if he could make an appointment to work individually on sexual and addictions issues. He has been in treatment with Dr. R for 3 years.

Dr. R described treatment as focusing on overcoming grief over his wife's passing, developing a healthy relationship with his adult daughters, and overcoming some habits he wanted to eliminate. Samuel drank wine approximately three times per week but had a goal of quitting altogether. He quit smoking cold turkey, as did his mother when she ended her snuff habit. Dr. R described his strengths as being authentic and honest with himself and others, being committed to his recovery group, and his Christian faith. His weaknesses were his loneliness and lack of flexibility—once he has chosen a course of action, he is reluctant to change it. While this can be positive, as in his smoking cessation, it has also had negative consequences for him. Dr. R's cognitive behavioral theoretical approach was employed to address Samuel's guilt, self-blame, grief, insecurity, and struggles to understand issues from a woman's perspective.

Dr. J saw Samuel during a period of approximately 6 weeks when Dr. R was not available. He was seen on a biweekly basis, as had been the case with Dr. R. His presenting concern to Dr. J was coping with a breakup with his girlfriend, "Deena," the prior month. She had said she "couldn't do it anymore." By that she meant that she could not deal with his demands for a more committed relationship because of the multiple strains of work and raising her young child. The impact of this loss prompted him to accept a referral for supportive treatment during Dr. R's absence.

Samuel met Deena on the job and had been involved with her for four months, though he'd known her for two years. Deena is 25 years younger than Samuel, a parallel to his own parents' age difference. Samuel says that she has been used to dealing with older men, as the fathers of both of her children are at least 10 years older than she. She was living with the father of the youngest. The living arrangement was not shared with Samuel in the beginning of their relationship and contributed to his sense of deception. The couple, like Samuel and his wife, had poor communication skills. Deena reportedly often took his comments to be corrective, critical, and condescending. He took hers to be manipulative, threatening, and sometimes demeaning. Each saw the other as controlling and attempted to gain dominance in the relationship.

At one point the couple considered marriage and living together, but Deena backed out just as Samuel was about to sign a lease on an apartment. It was at this point that he presented for treatment with Dr. J. It is significant to note that there had been sexual intimacy but no intercourse in their relationship. His faith prevented him from consummating the relationship, but he was comfortable with "everything but."

Samuel was deeply grieving what he feared was the demise of his "love" relationship (as it reemerged other losses—deaths of wife and mother). He was all but inconsolable and could not consider moving on. Dr. R had asked him to list the pros and cons of being involved with Deena, and he recognized that the cons outnumbered the pros by 50%, but he was not dissuaded. Among the cons was his perceived "addictive" need to be with her under any terms possible. When Dr. J referenced a cultural touchstone when she asked about his situation's similarity to Bill Withers's song "Use Me," he said that the song was on his playlist because it was an accurate description. One line of the lyrics talks about being used feeling so good as to be worth it (Withers, 1972). As noted by both Samuel and Dr. R, he persists even when it might not be in his best interest. He recognized the relationship's red flags from the beginning, for example, the requirement for surreptitious meetings and unpredictable meeting times, lack of affirming words, and ultimately the living arrangement (her living together partner considered them to be a family) but he would not, could not, let go. The conflict with his daughter over the suitability of their relationship has (note present tense) not deterred him. He suspected that the daughter was more concerned about a diminished inheritance than about protecting him. He said he was not willing to sacrifice his potential happiness to the daughter's selfish concerns.

Dr. J, also using a cognitive behavioral approach, focused their sessions on identifying coping skills (e.g., calling on his "persistence to success," or stubbornness), accessing supportive resources (e.g., leaning on his support group and leaning into his faith), and challenging his catastrophic predictions (e.g., making more logical and less emotional assessments of ultimate outcomes).

Multicultural Issues

Samuel indicated that he selected Dr. R on the basis of his initial impression of her warmth and approachability. He said he preferred working with a female (Samuel used the binary concept of male-female without reference to gender identity), as he had always been more comfortable talking about emotional issues with women. He shared with Dr. R that he often struggled with understanding a woman's perspective. Dr. J posed a question regarding whether either of his identities, being male or being Black, carried more meaning. He said being Black carried more due to the stresses of growing up Black in the rural south. Maleness was a benefit. He noted that he recognized that women are treated with less respect, adding that that was a bit surprising given that "we all have mothers."

Samuel denied that age was a factor in his selecting Dr. R, though she was 20 years his junior. He had seen a "younger" Black male therapist briefly in the past but found him to be incompatible because he talked too much about himself and seemed to "brag" about things, both of which Samuel found unacceptable to his religious beliefs. The honesty that Dr. R noted can be seen in his own admission that "God is not pleased" with much of his behavior either.

It is interesting to note that he referenced comparative age in relation to the Black male therapist. He also saw a Black female therapist in the late 1980s, whom he described as "older." Clearly age differences are recurrent and significant themes for him and should not be surprising given his life stage and fears of being alone—not having a mate for the rest of his life. The surprise may be in his lack of recognition of it.

Samuel stated that race was not a factor, believing that skill and empathy outweigh race in most situations. Neither Samuel nor Dr. R reported any difficulty or hesitation in addressing racial, cultural, or sociopolitical matters in the session. Several studies have shown that racial parity does not necessarily improve outcomes (Goode-Cross & Grim, 2016; Hayes et al., 2016). Samuel stated that these issues rarely come up as his focus is primarily on his personal, day-to-day issues. It may be argued that attention to cultural issues should be governed by their salience to the client (Hook et al., 2013); thus, Samuel's narrow focus on intrapersonal matters would allow the macro impact of racism to be contained. Perhaps he needed to prioritize allocation of his available psychic energy. It might also be argued that the insidiousness of systemic racism infects the psyche of people of color (living in the United States for certain) and, in a counter-transferential fashion, the psyche of majority race members as well. Must systemic racism be recognized, acknowledged, and called by its name in therapy? Some researchers say yes. Fuertes et al. (2002) believed that discussing race and racial differences early in treatment is requisite to cultural competence. However, as with most issues, timing is everything, and individuals vary in what they need.

Dr. R noted that she sees 10% to 20% African Americans in her private practice. As a rule, she introduces the topic of differences (e.g., race, gender, age) in the intake interview. She ascertains possible identity differences and opens up the conversation to consider any possible benefits/challenges/congruences her clients want to explore. Hook et al. (2013) reported on the importance of the therapist initiating those dialogues about race and culture as it reflects cultural humility, which, as previously noted, is a key component of multicultural competence. Dr. R initiated a discussion about their difference in terms of family structure. She explored whether Samuel thought her lack of personal familiarity with his extended family life experience might not allow her sufficient insight. She concluded that exploring this was indeed important in helping her understand the impact on his marriage, his current relationship, and sexual behaviors. This represents cultural humility in the therapist's recognition of knowledge gaps and willingness to learn from the patient about what their differences might signify.

For Samuel, faith compatibility was a far more salient factor in his preferences. His religious community regards affiliation as being a member of THE church. Its membership bestows a high level of kinship and "chosen" identity. Having such, Dr. R would have had "supercharged" credentials.

Research has consistently shown that Black Americans are more religious (church membership and attendance, devotional activities, frequency of prayer, use of religious resources in coping with life problems) than other racial groups (Gallup & Lindsay, 1999) across measures and across ages (Krause & Chatters, 2005; Levin et al., 1994; C. Smith et al., 2002; R. J. Taylor et al., 1996). When working with clients of color, particularly Black clients, who profess religious convictions, it is difficult to overstate the importance of not only unpacking the significance of them but also respecting, even utilizing, those convictions where possible.

Therapists, regardless of orientation, have sometimes been characterized as being antireligious (King-Spooner, 2001; Tummala-Narra, 2009). In a study assessing perceptions of patients about secular therapists, Cragun and Friedlander (2012) found that most clients reported positive experiences but poorer outcomes with therapists who were not perceived as open and willing to discuss religious beliefs. They suggested that the benefits of initiating discussions at intake about spiritual beliefs are reaped not only in creating a safe environment but also in setting the stage for full disclosure in other areas.

Given that Samuel was not aware of Dr. J's religious affiliation, she inquired about his decision to contact her. Religion, under most circumstances, would govern his selection. He stated that he was in such pain at the time that it did not even matter what Dr. J's religious affiliation was. He was in such a "bad place" that beyond getting help, not much else mattered.

Dr. J asked Samuel about other experiences and events that he recalled as prominent in "living while Black." (If this is not a readily understood concept, research and consultation are advised.) He reported that he has always been concerned about physical safety. He recalled a particular experience that stayed with him. One evening he'd missed his ride home from football practice and had to walk home a distance of about 20 miles. While walking along a two-lane highway in the dark, he thought he heard gunshots. He lay down in a ditch for about 30 minutes until the suspected danger was likely to have passed. He did not have the luxury of feeling safe from aggression and harassment by the authorities "in the south in the '60s." He feared being shot and knew that nothing would be done about it if he were! Given the current environment of the Black Lives Matter movement, Samuel may still have safety concerns. This should become a part of the therapy discourse when working with people of color, Black people especially.

Return to Treatment With Dr. R

As soon as Dr. R was available, Samuel returned to treatment with her. She was eager to explore what the therapy time with Dr. J had meant to him and to their relationship. Samuel described that it was helpful but that he had wanted to get back to the work they were doing. He was satisfied with the progress he was making with her and did not want to start over. As noted, he agreed to "bridge therapy" only because he was in so much pain.

Implications

Dr. R attributes the strength of their therapeutic alliance to a number of factors. She notes that her multicultural training and ongoing teaching on the subject greatly affected their work. Dr. R said,

> I have learned that we are much more effective when we notice—rather than ignore—our differences. It frees up communication so that we are both teaching and learning from one another. It minimizes possible perceived power inequities and increases trust and investment. It allows clients to come as they are rather than pretend and withhold information. It helps to eliminate stereotype threat. (personal communication, October 23, 2019)

Regarding the shared religious beliefs, Dr. R believes that it allowed her and Samuel to explore certain principles such as forgiveness, prayer, and Christ's love; but religion did not play as central a role in treatment as it has with some of her other clients. A more prominent theme in Samuel's treatment has been his desire for her to "hold him accountable" and help him accept more blame than she thought therapeutically warranted. Accountability and blame may have their roots in religious guilt, but Dr. R. focused on Samuel's expressed preference. She found it challenging but worked to facilitate an internal change rather than an external accountability.

Clearly, Samuel's religious belief was a highly significant feature of his cultural identity, yet we see that beyond the intake phase with Dr. R, it did not always loom large in his therapy. Religious similarity was not requisite in his willingness to work with Dr. J. This may have some significance for therapists who are fearful of addressing religion in treatment. The willingness to explore, appreciating what one may not believe, and allowing the client to determine the ebb and flow of therapeutic issues can allow the multicultural relationship to flourish. We don't have to be the same, but we do have to respect how we are different.

Both Dr. R and Dr. J initiated discussions about race. With both therapists Samuel denied having any current race-related issues he needed to address. Presuming he felt freer to discuss such issues with Dr. J because of phenotypic similarity, Cabral and Smith (2011) and Wintersteen et al. (2005) suggested that indeed that was the case. He endorsed that he was comfortable working with Dr. J, related historical information about racially charged experiences, and responded to culturally specific metaphors. These topics were initiated both by Samuel and Dr. J to be sure that neither the client nor the therapist was avoiding addressing important multicultural issues by attending to them *only if* they were brought up. This dual therapeutic contact provided an opportunity to validate the lack of avoidance.

Admittedly, a number of therapeutic issues surfaced in this case that have not been placed under the lens of the multicultural microscope: the relevance and influence of Samuel's "strong Black mother," dynamics of this relational power struggle and its rootedness in the parental dynamics (e.g., fear of, and attraction to, being controlled), the cultural implications of wide age variations in relationships, the intrapsychic costs of Black male safety vigilance, balancing faith and sexual intimacy, and much more. Not every important multicultural factor was relevant or could be covered if so.

At the 6-month follow-up, Samuel continued to participate in individual therapy with Dr. R and attend his support group. He indicated that he and Deena were thriving and anticipated getting married in 6 months. He was convinced that she loved him because she showed it. He deemed this as an affirmation that his stubbornness generally pays off. There had been only a mild thaw in the relationship with his daughters. He talked with them about what he needed in life and figured they will simply have to accept his choices. Dr. R documented the progress he reported.

It may be concluded that Dr. R's cultural humility allowed Samuel to explore what he needed and enabled her to comfortably refer him to another racially matched therapist that facilitated his return to their work together. Both agreed that her gender and manner may have prompted the initial contact, but it is her respect for all of Samuel's cultural identities that keeps him engaged.

This chapter addressed the therapeutic process and multicultural change process via the therapist–client relationship, common factors critical to the role of the therapist, and the role of the client. The case of Samuel elucidates some of these essential common factors as well as one way a multicultural therapeutic process was employed that resulted in effective change for this client. In the next chapter, we describe multiculturalism in education, training, and professional development.

Evaluation: Integrating Multiculturalism and Social Justice in Psychological Theories of Change

In this chapter, we evaluate multiple aspects of multicultural therapy, and we look at its limitations regarding range of applicability, especially given that individuals have multiple and intersecting identities. The chapter looks at how the predictions of its growth and impact are borne out by examining its infusion into the three foundational theoretical orientations and how its principles are woven into the fabric of training, competency evaluation, and assessment of professional preparedness. Expanding on the key concepts identified in the previous chapter, this chapter also takes up the issue of social justice as an ethical imperative in multicultural therapy. Use of individual case examples and broad cultural movements shows the micro- and macronecessity of employing a social justice lens to multicultural psychotherapy in particular and psychotherapy in general.

https://doi.org/10.1037/0000279-005
Multicultural Therapy: A Practice Imperative, by M. J. T. Vasquez and J. D. Johnson

In Chapter 2, we addressed how the history of multicultural therapy has come to be regarded as a "Fourth Force" following the three foundational theoretical orientations of psychodynamic, humanistic, and cognitive behaviorism. The question arises as to whether the major theoretical models, developed with Eurocentric foundations, are inherently unable to meet or respect the needs of individuals who do not, will not, cannot be treated under Eurocentric theoretical assumptions (Bhatia, 2002; Comas-Díaz & Torres Rivera, 2020; Poortinga, 1999). Roudinesco (1990) suggested that psychological science is "affected by the ideals of the society in which it was produced" (p. 175). Colonialism, characterized by Okazaki et al. (2008) as a specific form of oppression, permeated Eurocentric societies and philosophical thought when the earliest psychological theories and therapies were in their infancy. Using psychodynamic therapy as an example, Frosh (2013) reminded us that the history of psychoanalysis reflected "the colonial and racist (including antisemitic [sic]) assumptions prevalent in the Europe out of which psychoanalysis arose" (p. 143). Psychoanalytic language is replete with references like "primitive," describing not only the concept of a certain type of fantasy or behavior but also of cultures and mentality—a savage (primitive) versus a civilized mental life. Primitive, in such referents, is the "other," an inferior.

Some multicultural researchers (e.g., Koç & Kafa, 2019) question whether Eurocentric origin psychotherapy models can be culturally adapted, either by trying to align them with the needs of people of a particular country or culture or by aligning them with local psychotherapy models. Koç and Kafa (2019) argued that "Western-origin therapies themselves are local models" and questioned "whether it is possible to adapt a product of a specific culture to another" (p. 108). In spite of, or because of, these concerns, multicultural therapy has assumed a position of centrality from which other therapies are drawing. It can be argued that it is a force whose time has come given that the major theoretical models were inherently unable to meet the needs of culturally diverse individuals.

Researchers such as Fuertes et al. (2015) consider all therapeutic interactions to be inherently multicultural given that we are all socialized beings occupying unique social locations. Many therapists consider multicultural therapy to be a component of any effective therapy (Goodwin et al., 2018; Sehgal et al., 2011). Indeed, owing to its essential purpose, social justice character, and transtheoretical applications, multicultural therapy can be perceived as the epitome of professional practice.

Nearly 20 years ago, Norcross et al. (2002) surveyed psychotherapists of diverse theoretical backgrounds who predicted that the majority of psychotherapeutic orientations would have multicultural elements. Ten years later, Norcross et al. (2013) surveyed 70 psychotherapy experts for the purpose of forecasting trends in psychotherapy in the subsequent 10 years. They again predicted that employment of multicultural theories (also mindfulness, cognitive behavioral, and integrative theories) would increase the most.

There are clear points of congruence between multicultural theories and earlier theoretical systems. For example, assessing transference and countertransference issues in the psychodynamic tradition can be viewed by multiculturalists as recognizing and understanding that a patient's identity is fluid and multidetermined and that therapists' attitudes and beliefs influence clinical and empirical conceptualizations. Humanism's focus on establishing the alliance and viewing behavior in collective and social justice contexts (Comas-Díaz, 2012a) aligns with multicultural awareness and appreciation of individual and cultural differences. Behaviorism's consideration of learned behaviors and how the environment influences those behaviors is akin to the multicultural therapist's consideration of not only immediate environmental variables but also environmental influences in the larger context that includes analysis of available resources (P. A. Hays, 2009).

MULTICULTURAL THERAPY AND PSYCHODYNAMIC THERAPY

Even though quantitative and experimental data on psychodynamic therapy effectiveness in general are somewhat sparse, there have been some efforts to evaluate how well it lends itself to multicultural therapy.

The literature on ethnicity in psychodynamic therapy has demonstrated the need for therapists to be aware and knowledgeable of the cultural backgrounds of both themselves and their patients (Mishne, 2002; Summers, 2014).

For instance, Comas-Díaz and Jacobsen (1991) described the complexities of the fundamental psychoanalytic concepts of transference and countertransference in the multicultural dyad. They contended that, depending on the ethnic parity between patient and therapist, transference reactions can range from friendly to hostile, idealization to devaluation; countertransference reactions in dissimilar pairs are from "color-blindness" to aggression or from overidentification to distancing in ethnically similar pairs. They saw opportunities in the language of cultural transference and countertransference in helping therapists to understand themselves better and explore their own areas of cultural discomfort.

Tummala-Narra (2016) addressed cultural competence (a key element of multicultural therapy) in her book, *Psychoanalytic Theory and Cultural Competence in Psychotherapy*. That book is regarded as a comprehensive, clearly written, clinically relevant discourse on cultural competence from a psychoanalytic perspective (Gaztambide, 2018). Tummala-Narra addressed a broad range of overlapping concepts, including the critical importance of recognizing the client's and therapist's indigenous cultural narratives. In identifying the areas of overlap, she emphasized the essentiality of therapist self-examination in shaping what is heard in therapy, noted the development of new psychoanalytic diversity-oriented language, and attended to the impact of social oppression and cultural attitudes toward race in social identity development. She also provided a historical overview and acknowledged the history of psychoanalytic neglect of sociocultural issues.

According to Fuertes et al. (2015), an example of transference in multicultural therapy may be a situation in which the therapist is perceived or unconsciously experienced as an oppressor or as a representative of an unjust system. They suggested that these reactions may stem from actual past experiences of hurt or fear that need airing within the session. Fuertes et al. (2015) thus advised that the reactions by both therapist and client should be examined and worked through empathically, and they noted that countertransference in multicultural therapy may occur when the therapist retreats or withdraws psychologically, even briefly, out of their own discomfort or anxiety when their client expresses affect and cognitions related to their experiences with racism, bias, and/or oppression.

One of the authors of this book, Dr. J, recalls a countertransference reaction when she temporarily retreated when her client made a statement she perceived as a microaggression. Dr. J was working with a White woman who had left her marriage and family to be in a relationship with a Black man. She was exploring her decisions and their ramifications, not only the conflict and estrangement from her adult children but also the financial consequences. She described her Black male paramour as "n****r rich." Dr. J was momentarily stunned at the phrase, in part because she was not sure of its meaning, but she presumed it was not complimentary. The patient did not notice the therapist's withdrawal and continued with her narrative. After recovering, Dr. J was conflicted about returning to explore the point as she was uncertain whose need it met to do so at the time. Take a moment to consider what you would do in this instance. In a subsequent session, Dr. J attempted to address both her own reaction and explore the patient's awareness of the "microaggression." She told the patient that she had been surprised to hear the term (after researching its meaning: the stereotype portraying Black people as having money in their pockets and none in the bank). She asked if the patient could see that such a phrase would be offensive to the therapist and other Black people. The patient expressed some surprise and indicated that she would avoid use of the term in the future.

The research literature contains case examples of the application of multicultural theory in psychoanalytic therapy. Vazquez (2014), for instance, reported that in an examination of three therapeutic dyads involving women of color, both psychoanalytic and multicultural conceptualizations were important in the healing process. The therapists' shared relational processes were examined in relation to multicultural concepts such as racial and ethnic identity development, acculturation, and colorism. The inclusion of these concepts had a significant impact on understanding how discriminatory and traumatic experiences affected their clients of color throughout their lives.

In their study of a large Asian population's use of defense mechanisms, a key psychoanalytic concept, Tori and Bilmes (2002) determined that psychoanalytic psychology has multicultural and contemporary relevance. They examined the unconscious, self-protective coping among Thais and posited that their test of defense mechanisms was able to distinguish groups with known psychosocial differences and concluded that "psychoanalytic defense conceptualizations have broad cross-cultural applicability" (p. 717).

Rodriguez et al. (2008) described a psychodynamic therapy case study where cultural issues were uncovered and addressed using the psychodynamic tool of parallel process. A number of key cultural concepts came into focus in the treatment of a 38-year-old Hispanic woman by a Hispanic female therapist. Therapy addressed how cultural similarities and dissimilarities enhanced and hindered treatment. Use of the parallel process, where the therapist-in-training recreates, or parallels, the client's problems by way of relating to her own supervisor, brought an additional layer of analytic scrutiny. It allowed the supervisor to highlight the therapist's transference and countertransference issues (e.g., avoiding addressing negative maternal transference, demonstrations of closeness, or being Spanish "enough" or poor "enough"). The case demonstrated the integration of multicultural and psychodynamic modalities.

Giving credit to feminist ideology and multicultural psychology for challenging psychoanalysis's characterization of religion as pathological, Tummala-Narra (2009) contended that psychoanalysis and religion share a goal of identity elucidation and specifically addressed how religion and spiritual beliefs influence identity development. In a case study of a biracial (African American and White American) Christian woman, Tummala-Narra, an Indian American Hindu woman, recounted how a relational psychoanalytic perspective allowed them to explore religion and spirituality in a respectful, nonpathologizing way. Further, the therapist's ability to confront her own fears of losing objectivity or altering the power dynamic in their relationship by exposing information about her own spiritual life allowed for a more open and authentic engagement with the client.

Berger et al. (2014) noted that Asian Americans and Pacific Islanders, compared with other ethnic populations, were least likely to utilize mental health services and wondered if the underutilization was due to the scarcity of culturally competent providers. They questioned whether previous work on multicultural competencies was generalizable from university-based trainees and staff to community mental health providers. They conducted a study assessing 221 Los Angeles County community mental health clinicians' characteristics, their theoretical orientations, and cultural competency and found that psychodynamic or humanistic orientations correlated with poorer multicultural counseling relationships (e.g., therapists adhering to those theoretical orientations who worked with minority clients were less able to perceive that their race caused clients to mistrust them) and a lower level of community awareness, than did therapists with an eclectic or behavioral (e.g., cognitive behavioral or behavior modification) orientation. They did find, however, that community knowledge (e.g., how well the therapist was able to describe the communities of color in the service area) mediated multicultural awareness between therapeutic orientations. The authors suggested that there are opportunities for (psychodynamic and humanistic) therapists to develop more cultural awareness and improve their relationships with ethnic minority clients by becoming more involved with diverse populations in their communities.

Adlerian theory and therapy exemplify the junction of psychodynamic and multicultural concepts particularly well. The Adlerian approach to treatment emphasizes the social embeddedness of human beings, seeing personal problems within a sociocultural context. Goals of Adlerian therapy focus on empowering client decisions about change and, like multicultural therapy, deals with the individual and the family. Of note is the lasting impact on culturally diverse populations reflected in *Brown v. Board of Education* in 1954. Kenneth B. Clark and other social scientists cited Adlerian theory in their successful argument against the separate but equal doctrine that defended school segregation (Irby, 2013).

MULTICULTURAL THERAPY AND HUMANISM

There was a time when humanism did not fully live out its creed of emphasizing "contextual dimensions" in addressing clients' reflections on their relationship with self, others, and the larger psychosocial world. The clarion call for increased diversity in humanistic psychology was sounded as far back as the mid-20th century when existential philosopher Paul Tillich (1957) famously stated that

> the citizens of a city are not guilty of the crimes committed in their city, but they are guilty participants in the destiny of [humanity] as a whole and in the destiny of their city in particular; for their acts in which freedom was united with destiny have contributed to the destiny in which they participated. (p. 59)

Hoffman et al. (2015) warned that failure to help humanistic psychology become more multiculturally sensitive would deem it "guilty of contributing to the perpetuation of a culturally insensitive psychology" (p. 52). Though progress was noted, Hoffman et al. advised that satisfaction with that level of progress was unacceptable—humanistic psychology should take advantage of the energy flow and "transform humanistic psychology into a mature multicultural approach to psychology" (p. 52).

Schneider and Längle (2012) regarded multicultural therapy and humanism as integral to one another. Comas-Díaz (2012a) argued that multiculturalism embraces humanistic values, for example, collective and social justice contexts. She noted that "the multicultural–humanistic connection is a necessary shift in the evolution of psychotherapy" (p. 437) and that multicultural traditions have historically provided humanistic ways of shaping identity, agency, and freedom. She specifically identified contextualism, which Hurtado (2010) described as therapists attending to their clients' perspectives rather than imposing their own interpretive voice; holism, including the patient's subjective experience of illness in the diagnosis and treatment; and liberation (consolidating identity by healing the split between the relational self and the environment) as multicultural–humanistic constructs that help patients derive self-meaning.

Felder and Robbins (2016) acknowledged that phenomenology and humanistic psychology do not appear to have adequately referenced the significance of sociocultural contexts in daily life. They posited a mindfulness and meditative sociocultural existential psychotherapy approach that integrates the mindfulness meditation (which predates the mindfulness-based cognitive behavioral third wave) with sociocultural constructs and suggested that such an approach creates a greater sense of wholeness for the patient as a sociocultural being.

The field of transpersonal psychology is often regarded as closely related to or an outgrowth of humanistic psychology; indeed, one of its better-known pioneers was the famous humanistic psychologist Abraham Maslow (Lattuada, 2018; S. Taylor, 2015). Definitions vary, but most include referents to higher potential, beyond ego, and other spiritual elements. After analyzing 35 years of publications, Hartelius et al. (2007) acknowledged that transpersonal psychology has had "difficulty defining itself" (p. 1). Walsh and Vaughan (1993) offered this definition of the *transpersonal*: "experiences in which the sense of identity or self extends beyond (trans) the individual or personal to encompass wider aspects of humankind, life, psyche or cosmos" (p. 203). The kinship between transpersonal psychology, a humanistic psychology, and multicultural psychology is seen in their sharing of concepts such as spirituality and other states of awareness as honoring the values and potential of the individual. Hartelius et al. (2007) recognized that the ego is contextualized and thus must be considered within the interrelations of community, social history, and the environment. Those authors also saw transpersonal psychology as having a liberation psychology imperative (i.e., to oppose growing religious and cultural alienation, theories of intellectual inferiority of races, genders, and classes). They described a future in which transpersonal psychology

> offers the vision of a truly inclusive psychology that spans the many forms of human diversity—a psychology that opposes specious justifications for oppression of any person or group. It challenges the egoic view that truth is possessed by the society most effective at disposing of its rivals. Instead, it offers a holistic and transformative vision in which authentic meaning can be shared by all of humanity. (p. 153)

There are areas of divergence between multicultural and humanistic therapies. Humanism has historically affirmed the individual's ability and responsibility to lead ethical lives of personal fulfillment that aspire to the greater good (American Humanistic Association, n.d.). This philosophy may contradict the collectivist "live in harmony" concept typically ascribed to multicultural approaches. Despite difficulties with conceptual clarity and the potential for greater stereotyping of culturally diverse groups (Wong et al., 2018), individualism versus collectivism is often identified as a central point of divergence between U.S. societal values and racial and ethnic group values. Wong et al. (2018) urged caution in the use of the collectivism-individualism dichotomy in the study of culture, noting the lack of conceptual clarity and the potential for greater stereotyping of culturally diverse groups.

When therapeutic orientations, among other variables, were associated with cultural competency by Los Angeles County mental health clinician–researchers (Berger et al., 2014), results showed a difference between nonbehavioral and eclectic/behavioral orientations. The latter reported a higher level of community knowledge than the nonbehavioral (psychodynamic and humanistic) therapists. Community awareness facilitated multicultural skills. The inference to be drawn is that humanistic therapists should become more personally involved with diverse communities, thereby improving their perceptions of having better relationships with ethnic minority clients.

MULTICULTURAL THERAPY AND COGNITIVE BEHAVIOR THERAPY

Cognitive behavior therapy is most often referenced in relation to multicultural therapy. Sharing a number of basic premises (P. A. Hays, 2009), both orientations emphasize the need to adapt therapeutic interventions to the unique circumstances of the individual in therapy. Both additionally emphasize the empowerment of clients as well as the therapeutic aspects of clients' strengths, resilience, and support systems. The integration of multicultural therapy and behavioral therapy has been explored in a number of books and articles covering a variety of conditions and situations. For example, Diaz-Martinez et al. (2010) examined how cognitive behavioral, feminist, and multicultural approaches were influential in treating migration-related stress in a suicidal patient.

With its emphasis on evidence-based practice, cognitive behavior therapy's integration with multicultural therapy's focus on cultural competence expands both the relevance and effectiveness of psychotherapy. Efforts to provide specific training suggestions for integrating multicultural competencies into cognitive behavior therapy for mental health professionals are highlighted in the significant contributions of Pamela A. Hays (2009), who identified 10 multicultural concepts that should be considered in the provision of cognitive behavior therapy:

1. Assess the person's and family's needs with an emphasis on culturally respectful behavior.
2. Identify culturally related strengths and supports.
3. Clarify what part of the problem is primarily environmental (i.e., external to the client) and what part is cognitive (internal) with attention to cultural influences.
4. For environmentally based problems, focus on helping the client to make changes that minimize stressors, increase personal strengths and supports, and build skills for interacting more effectively with the social and physical environment.
5. Validate clients' self-reported experiences of oppression.
6. Emphasize collaboration over confrontation, with attention to client-therapist differences.
7. With cognitive restructuring, question the helpfulness (rather than the validity) of the thought or belief.
8. Do not challenge core cultural beliefs.
9. Use the client's list of culturally related strengths and supports to develop a list of helpful cognitions to replace the unhelpful ones.
10. Develop weekly homework assignments with an emphasis on cultural congruence and client direction. (pp. 356–358)

In spite of these cultural adaptations, behavioral therapy, and in particular, cognitive behavior therapy, may not always be compatible with multicultural therapy. P. A. Hays (2019) cautioned that attributing a client's distress to intrapersonal issues only (e.g., faulty cognitions) while failing to consider environmental contributions not only puts undue onus on the client but also may suggest that the environment is acceptable. Further, they asserted that a singular approach could cause treatment to be ineffective. It is incumbent upon the therapist to perceive and maintain a balanced perspective regarding the relative contributions of cognitive problems and the oppressive environmental systems that spawn or maintain them. It is not just what and how one thinks that is the source of distress. We must also consider the environment that may contribute to distress.

LIMITATIONS OF MULTICULTURAL THERAPY

The foregoing discussion sought to identify areas of congruence and convergence between multicultural theories and earlier theoretical systems. An exploration of limitations should bring up the issue of evidence. The principal tenets of multicultural therapy have intuitive validity, but what is the evidence of effectiveness? T. B. Smith and Trimble (2016), giving a nod to the American Psychological Association, Task Force on Evidence-Based Practice (2006), emphasized that "a solid research foundation is essential to the credibility and long-term effectiveness of multicultural guidelines for practitioners" (p. 4). Given the increasing scholarship on the subject and to address criticisms of unproven generalizations, they conducted a meta-analysis of 215 published studies encompassing several ethnic groups involving more than 50,000 participants. Their research data supported a number of implications for practitioners, including that

- therapists benefit from multicultural competence education;
- people of color underutilize mental health services (particularly Asian Americans) and are at greater risk for early termination (particularly African Americans);
- clinicians should be attuned to levels of acculturation and client perceptions and should empower clients reporting racist encounters; and
- clinicians should become the learner in understanding their own and the client's worldviews (p. 247).

Even with its transtheoretical applications, does multicultural therapy work for everyone? One can certainly argue that it should, given that we are all multicultural beings; all therapy, therefore, is intrinsically multicultural. Are there, nevertheless, limitations or restrictions to its application? The authors have not identified any research showing that multicultural therapy as an approach is inappropriate for any person, group, condition, or location. In fact, it is perhaps the most universally applicable system. There may, however, be some situations or circumstances that do not lend themselves to unambiguous application of multicultural principles as described in the examples that follow.

Assignment of cases to therapists on a rotating basis in public systems (e.g., community mental health centers, university counseling centers) can be challenging from a multicultural or social justice perspective. There may not be a clear multicultural directive when "Conviction of Conscience" issues arise, as in the Julea Ward case, where a counseling trainee refused to see specific clients on the basis of religious beliefs (Behnke, 2013). Specifically, Ward refused to counsel a gay client as part of her training; the university determined that this was discrimination and expelled Ward from the program. She sued, claiming she was being singled out for her religious beliefs. The university chose to settle with Ward and agreed to pay her $75,000 but did not admit any wrongdoing nor change any of its policies. Conversely, what does it mean when a patient who presents for treatment refuses service from certain therapists? We often try to accommodate gender preferences, but what of other preferences? What is the prevailing wisdom? If one were working with patients whose treatment goals are antithetical to multicultural principles (e.g., White supremacists or "incels," members of an online subculture who are mostly male, heterosexual, and White, and are "involuntarily celibate," though desiring, are unable to find a romantic or sexual partner)? An interesting ethical question might be, is it the responsibility of the therapist to treat such persons, showing fidelity to the multicultural principle of inclusion, or refuse to treat as it may be seen as empowering the person to continue on a socially destructive path? It seems ethically appropriate that if a therapist judges differences to be too large to traverse effectively, then one should refer.

We can look at "limitations" from another viewpoint. Multicultural therapy has not been shown to be inappropriate, but there are studies showing that it has not been more effective than other systems in terms of outcome. Tao et al. (2015) employed traditional measures of therapeutic processes and outcomes, that is, working alliance, client satisfaction, general counseling competence, session impact, and symptom improvement, in assessing client ratings of therapist multicultural competencies. Results of their meta-analysis did not find any significant correlations between multicultural competence and outcome. They further noted some evidence of publication bias with published studies showing larger effect sizes than unpublished dissertations. In another study, Owen et al. (2011) examined the relationship between clients' assessment of their therapist's multicultural competence to determine if higher ratings were associated with therapy outcomes. They found that multicultural competencies did not account for the variability in therapy outcomes; neither the client's nor the therapist's race was associated with patients' perceptions.

Culturally or racially matched dyads have been believed to facilitate understanding and acceptance, providing a kind of multicultural shorthand for communication. Outcomes, however, have been mixed, as noted. Consideration should be given to the potential barriers that can be created. Matching may obscure issues within the therapist (Rodriguez et al., 2008) that can affect the treatment. The therapist of color has lived with the same sociopolitical realities as the patient. Does the patient trigger feelings of stereotype threat in the therapist or vice versa? Stereotype threat is a phenomenon when an individual perceives risk of confirming a negative stereotype about one's group (Steele & Aronson, 1995). Differences in socioeconomic level or education may counteract the presumed benefits of similarity. The therapist who has grown up in a resource-rich environment may not be aware of their internalized implicit bias when treating patients from lower socioeconomic statuses. It may prove difficult to empathize with a client who utilizes social welfare benefits. Conversely, a therapist who has struggled to overcome an impoverished childhood may experience empathy failure with patients who may be perceived as "the one percent" (i.e., those who are wealthy). There are a number of areas of privilege that can go unacknowledged or unpacked (McIntosh, 1988) within matched therapist–patient dyads. Being Christian, heterosexual, well-educated, able-bodied, and/or male are advantages in U.S. society that can negatively affect psychotherapy if those privileges remain unexamined and unconscious.

The charge that multicultural therapy focuses too exclusively on racial and ethnic minorities (Ratts & Pedersen, 2014) has been made. Lowe and Mascher (2001) argued that cultural competence discussions frequently focus on race and ethnicity and advocated for inclusion of biases against gay, lesbian, bisexual, and transgender clients in models of cultural competence. Silverstein (2006) remarked that "multiculturalism has generally been narrowly defined in terms of race/ethnicity, overlooking the intersections of other aspects of diversity, such as class, gender, and sexual orientation" (p. 22). Search engines turn up comparatively much less published scholarship examining multicultural therapy or competence and other areas of identity, for example, spirituality or socioeconomic status.

Limitations of multicultural therapy are sometimes associated more with the therapist than the therapy. Multicultural therapy implies a well-trained therapist. Facility with terminology, having had "the" course, or being a member of a minority group does not qualify one as a culturally responsive professional. Multicultural competence is a continuous or lifelong endeavor that requires assertive commitment to growth. Furthermore, if a therapist is culturally proficient in working with members of one group, this does not suggest that they are competent to deliver effective services to other groups. We also know that some people, therapists included, are unable or unwilling to renounce their prejudice and privilege. In two independent studies, researchers found that, based on names, wording, and accents, therapists were less likely to offer appointments to Black callers leaving voicemail requests than White callers (Kugelmass, 2016; Shin et al., 2016). There's no certainty that training in multicultural competence will overcome ingrained prejudices.

Do we really know how to become competent? Ridley, Sahu, et al. (2021) challenged the entire multicultural movement to reconsider competence. That there is a substantial body of published scholarship on multicultural counseling competence attests to the power and promise of the movement, but it also reveals its fault lines. The writers maintained that the construct of competence lacks a cohesive "GPS"—a clear conceptualization of the journey, the destination, and the outlooks on the way to the destination. They contended that multicultural counseling competence is at an impasse; it is a construct in search of operationalization. Practitioners seeking clear direction as to how to reach therapeutic change, the ultimate purpose of multicultural counseling, are frustrated by the absence of maps and directional road signs. Ridley, Sahu, et al. (2021) listed 10 definitional problems that have brought the evolution of the construct to an impasse. The list covers an indistinct purpose, culturally general/culturally specific divide, terminology interchange, confusing competency with competence, lack of integration, no definition, ambiguity, equivocation, circular reasoning, and divergence. These valid concerns perhaps should factor in a viewpoint described by Goodwin et al. (2018) that multicultural competence may be a skill that is not stable and fixed. They offered that it may be fluid, not stably maintained, and varying across patient dyads. Flexibility in responsivity may be appropriate in certain patient contexts.

Ridley, Sahu, et al. (2021) also examined Huey et al.'s (2014) classification of the numerous models' multicultural competence into the three categories of skills-based, adaptation, and process-oriented models. They concluded that all three models suffer from a lack of prescriptive specificity about how to intervene, having only a surface incorporation of culture, and oversimplifying the multiple and interacting components. Ridley, Mollen, et al. (2021) identified the need for an integrated model that includes the strengths of all three. Their model has three phases covering intake through termination; five clinical operations, one of which is described as "deep structure incorporation of culture"; and processes focused on developing alliances and adapting interventions among others (Pope et al., 2021; Ridley, Mollen, et al., 2021). The model shows great promise as they predict in "advancing from the description of abstract competencies to the prescription of concrete actions, specifying what level of incorporation of culture qualifies as competent, elucidating the model's complexity, designing the model more representatively and researching its utility" (Ridley, Mollen, et al., 2021, p. 526).

INTERSECTIONALITIES

Intersectionality perhaps should be considered while discussing limitations of multicultural therapy. The intricacies of clients' and therapists' multiple identities confronting, conflicting, concealing, conflating, and/or coalescing, conjoining, cohering, or conforming creates a pattern too complex to be taught or mastered. Yet it remains a reality that they must be addressed despite the difficulties in doing so. One of the challenges is that multicultural competencies in research and practice tend to focus on one sociocultural identity at a time: race, ability, sexual orientation, religion, or privilege. No individual is single-faceted; each has interconnecting identities. Researchers such as D. W. Sue and Sue (2016) have pointed out that the plausibility of articulating and measuring MCCs (multicultural competencies)—especially skills and knowledge—for the entirety of a client's salient and less salient identities becomes untenable. Each aspect of identity carries emotional and political significance of culture, including differential power and status (Walker, 2020).

The challenge for the multicultural therapist is in attaining multiple competencies in regard to the varied identities each person carries. Walker (2020) described intersectionality as carrying many cultures in one body. For example, if a Muslim woman who recently emigrated from Lebanon, is lesbian identified, and has scoliosis requiring a wheelchair presents for treatment for anxiety, what competency skills does the therapist need and where does one begin? Is it a possible or reasonable expectation that any therapist should be able to demonstrate competency in all her identities? The short answer is "of course not," but how do we focus our work?

Our definition of evidence-based practice might reasonably inform that question, for in addition to having familiarity with the relevant scholarship in the areas identified, and using one's clinical skills, the patient's preferences and priorities must be considered. As the case study shared in Chapter 3 suggests, the patient's hierarchy of concerns should dictate the focus of treatment. This, however, potentially leaves unaddressed issues that the patient might be unaware of or is avoiding. A skilled multicultural therapist would experiment to determine which aspects of identity are at the forefront of the psychotherapy, and what aspects might be brought to the forefront for the benefit of the client, based on their needs.

Silverstein (2006) argued that the intersection of multiculturalism and feminism are bidirectionally challenging, writing that "multiculturalism has focused almost exclusively on race and ethnicity, whereas feminism has focused for the most part on White, middle-class women" (p. 21). Preferring one identity over the other fails to recognize their intertwined roots in social justice as the "focus on a single domain, rather than the intersectionality of multiple domains, has contributed to the marginalization of both" (p. 22).

L. S. Brown (2009) has given significant consideration to intersectionalities. She first did so from her early scholarship on feminist therapy and then to her recognition of the centrality of cultural competence to effective psychotherapy. She pointed out that the etic—the general body of knowledge about a particular culture or group—and the emic—within-group perspectives—coupled with the therapists' acknowledgment of their own biases (and relinquishing the notion of objectivity) still might miss the competency mark. She argued that one must consider "self-invention," what the patient self-constructs or creates of their identities in the context of experiences of powerlessness and hopelessness. It is through the examination of intersectionalities that core concepts and critical experiences are disentangled, and more functional pathways are able to be identified.

SPIRITUALITY

The historical relationship between psychology and religion or spirituality has not always been mutually respectful. For example, Cherry (2020) cited from Freud's 1930 book, *Civilization and Its Discontents*, where he described religion as an "embarrassing product of humanity" and "patently infantile." Albert Ellis, founder of rational emotive behavioral therapy, in his pamphlet *The Case Against Religion: A Psychotherapist's View and the Case Against Religiosity* (1980), called religion pernicious, charged it with creating anxiety and hostility, and determined it to be a neurosis. Even the creator of the best-known form of humanistic therapy, person-centered therapy, Carl Rogers, was said to have died an atheist (Flannagan, 2018). He and other humanistic therapists may have found religious beliefs to be compatible with person-centered therapy except where doctrine is judgmental. There is still reparative work to be done.

That religion and spirituality are recognized as key elements of identity is due largely to developments in the multicultural therapy movement (Davis et al., 2020; Winkeljohn Black et al., 2021). Research has shown that adapting treatment to a patient's religious or spiritual beliefs results in greater improvements in their psychological and spiritual functioning compared with providing no treatment or not including religion and spirituality (Captari et al., 2018). The effective multicultural therapist seeks to understand the significance of religion not as evidence of pathology, though pathological religiosity can be present, but as a source of support within the individual and from the community. Training, however, has not kept pace. A number of articles have reported on the absence of preparation on how to incorporate religion and spirituality in psychotherapy (Oxhandler & Pargament, 2018; Winkeljohn Black et al., 2021).

How, then, does one acquire the needed competence? Barnett and Johnson (2011) proposed the following decision-making model about how and when to address spiritual and religious matters with the patient:

- Respectfully assess the client's religious or spiritual beliefs and preferences.
- Carefully assess any connection between the presenting problem and religious or spiritual beliefs and commitments.
- Weave the results of this assessment into the informed consent process.
- Honestly consider your countertransference to the client's religiousness.
- Honestly evaluate your competence in this case.

- Consult with experts in the area of religion and psychotherapy.
- If appropriate, clinically indicated, and the client gives consent, consult with the client's own clergy or other religious professional.
- Make a decision about treating the client or making a referral.
- Assess outcomes and adjust plan accordingly. (pp. 159–161)

Consider this brief vignette of 20-year-old Nadia, who presented for therapy with concerns about her relationship with her 23-year-old boyfriend. She questioned his fidelity in the relationship as he continued to maintain a close "friendship" with his ex-girlfriend. Her anxiety was fueled by the fact that she had made the decision to be intimate with him without being married. This clearly stood in opposition to her Islamic faith. Nadia still lived at home with her family while enrolled in a very good university and was doing well academically. Her boyfriend was not her parents' choice for a suitable suitor, and she was often tense about their fairly open dislike of him. Nadia denied being ambivalent about her sexual decisions but did not share them with her parents. Having had little dating experience, she worried a great deal that she couldn't trust her boyfriend and would get hurt as the parents had predicted.

The therapist's historic and current religious identification is Christian/Protestant. It is an important part of her identity. The therapy occurred in an area of the country where there is a significant Middle Eastern presence allowing for a fair amount of familiarity with Muslim customs. The therapist has treated Muslims before in her practice. The therapist wants to create a safe atmosphere in which Nadia can explore her trust issues.

Taking direction from the Barnett and Johnson (2011) model, we can begin assessing and addressing key multicultural considerations in Nadia's presentation. However, before employing a decision model, it is important to bring up the thorny issue of whether and when to address patient/therapist differences. This is an important consideration whether it pertains to race, religion, gender attractionality, or other identity aspect. Kuo (2021) recommended that multicultural differences be acknowledged at the beginning of treatment. He offered the following example of how to begin:

I am not a person of Muslim faith; how do you feel about working with me as your psychologist? As we work together, I would like to invite you to do the following if there are things about your faith or your Islamic identity that you feel I should understand; please let me know and bring it up to me so that I can talk about it. This is because cultural factors including religion and faith are very important for me in really understanding you and your experiences or problems. Does that sound OK with you?

Selecting some parts of the Barnett and Johnson (2011) model, we might consider the following:

- Respectfully assess the client's religious or spiritual beliefs and preferences.

    Ask open-ended questions about the significance of Islam for Nadia and her family. Even though religion is an important cultural identity that should be explored, the therapist must let Nadia determine what is most salient for her at the time. The presenting problem may just be what feels easy or safe to start with.

- Carefully assess any connection between the presenting problem and religious or spiritual beliefs and commitments.

    The fact that she is "dating" would likely pose a problem for dedicated adherents to the faith. "Courting" would be sanctioned, but dating would not. Explore the parents' objection to the boyfriend and the meaning of Nadia's choosing him.

- Honestly consider your countertransference to the client's religiousness.

    The therapist must explore her values regarding Islam. The therapist must ask herself what she has heard and what she believes about Islam. We are all filters for what we see and hear, particularly as regards media. Some biases are not filtered out. Does her interpretation of her Christianity have a value judgment regarding premarital sex?

- Honestly evaluate your competence in this case.

    The therapist feels fairly confident about her competence. Even though the therapist has had experience in treating Muslims and lives in a diverse area, it does not confer competence. The therapist may have some knowledge about the Muslim way of life but should understand that awareness and skills are also essential components of competence (Pedersen, 2002).

- Consult with experts in the area of religion and psychotherapy.
    The therapist should also commit to continuous learning through consultations (perhaps with Muslim therapists), continuing education, exploring firsthand experiences such as visiting a mosque, cultural celebrations, etc.

The culturally humble multicultural therapist views religion and spirituality as possible sources of interpersonal and intrapersonal strength. They are also worthy of exploration because they might elucidate other therapeutic issues. Cultural humility undergirds the multicultural therapist's approach to understanding a patient's religious beliefs or practices and presents an openness to learn from the patient as teacher. In an exquisite moment of learning, Dr. J asked a former patient how therapy facilitates spiritual growth/freedom or faith. During treatment, the patient made the epiphanous decision to pursue ministry training. Her reply was, "It's this process launched with a trusted therapist who holds a safe, encouraging space which opened me to a hunger for God who is the Deep and the Life Under All Lives" (personal communication, June 4, 2021).

The crossroads of multicultural therapy and gender individualities (expression, identity, sexual and romantic attraction) are well established, but some may argue that they are not necessarily well traveled. A concern is raised that the primary focus on race and ethnicity has obscured research on sexual orientation and gender identity minorities (Love et al., 2015; Moodley & Palmer, 2014; Ratts & Pedersen, 2014). The psychotherapist hoping to provide effective treatment with sexual minorities must factor in the added impact of discrimination. That it is associated with poorer health (Bogart et al., 2018) should not be surprising given the chronic stress associated with discrimination in the workplace, in the eyes of the law, by executive order, in religious institutions, and in society in general. Van Den Bergh (2004) believed that to become a culturally proficient therapist working with LGBTQ patients, one must understand the importance of safety in the workplace and the critical need for protection, inclusion, and equity in the workplace.

There are numerous areas of identity, visible and invisible, that intersect: (Dis)ability, language, immigration status, biraciality, colorism, age, size, literacy, and trauma history, among others, form and inform how we exist in the world. Even the most gifted multicultural therapist cannot be expert in addressing all of these identities. Nevertheless, we have an obligation to know what we don't know, grow where we need to grow, and be self-aware enough to know when we need to refer.

SOCIAL JUSTICE WORK AS AN ETHICAL IMPERATIVE IN MULTICULTURAL THERAPY

"A Safe Place to Land," a song by Sara Bareilles and John Legend (Bareilles & McKenna, 2019), asks the listener to envision how stressful it would be to be told not to move while standing in a burning building. That is what multicultural therapy would be asked to do without factoring in social justice considerations. How can we treat multicultural individuals without attending to the environmental conflagration that often surrounds them? The best individual therapy in the world cannot be so without recognizing that the individual also exists in a world outside the office and that they bring that world into the office. Can we sit and receive those narratives without the creation of imperative action? If we truly care about our clients and society's injustice, it is vitally important that we find ways to engage in social justice.

There are myriad definitions of social justice that address power dynamics (Ratts & Pedersen, 2014), advocate for sociopolitical reform (Thrift & Sugarman, 2019), and argue for "treating individuals equitably and fostering fairness and equality" (American Counseling Association, 2014, p. 3). In this monograph, we define *social justice* as "the goal to decrease human suffering and to promote human values of equality and justice" (Vasquez, 2012, p. 337). It is fortified by Thrift and Sugarman's (2019) ideology that "psychological services that merely help individuals adjust to circumstances of poverty and inequality, without doing anything to change these conditions, is a disservice to social justice" (p. 14).

Social justice in psychotherapy has been evolving as a value in psychology for decades (Leong et al., 2017; M. J. T. Vasquez, 2012). The American Psychological Association has made efforts to address human rights and social justice issues through its task force reports, guidelines, and policies. Specific issues addressed have included diversity and underrepresentation of minority group members and perspectives, women's issues, immigration and refugee concerns, concerns for those with disabilities, and rights of the LGBTQ community, among others. Social justice issues with a health perspective have included AIDS, obesity, and violence. Several of the APA guidelines have focused on identities that have been marginalized in society, including race and ethnicity, sexual orientation, women and girls, people with disabilities, older adults, and those with low-income and economic marginalization (see Introduction, this monograph). The APA's (2017a) *Ethical Principles of Psychologists and Code of Conduct* is a prime example of the association's commitment to and support of social justice. Its Preamble requires psychologists to "respect and protect civil and human rights"; Principle A: Beneficence and Nonmalfeasance urges "psychologists seek to safeguard the welfare and rights of those with whom they interact professionally and other affected persons"; Principle B: Fidelity and Responsibility states that psychologists should be "aware of their professional and scientific responsibilities to society and to the specific communities in which they work"; and perhaps most germanely, Principle D: Justice implores psychologists to "recognize that fairness and justice entitle all persons to access to and benefit from the contributions of psychology and to equal quality in the processes, procedures, and services being conducted by psychologists."

In response to the growing call for social justice and the ascendance of multicultural counseling, the American Counseling Association (ACA; 2003) developed a set of *Advocacy Competencies* to facilitate counselors' skills in assisting clients to overcome barriers that transcend the confines of the office. Those competencies include, among others, Student/Client Advocacy, Systems Advocacy, and Social/Political Advocacy and integrate the dimensions of advocacy done with the client and on behalf of the client. They encourage environmental interventions; exerting systems-change leadership at the school, organization, or community level; and use as exemplars "writing advocacy briefings regarding an issue, invitations to testify at hearings, appearing in mass media (e.g., talk shows, podcasts) to raise awareness of issues, and other actions where the counselor speaks on behalf of an issue" (ACA, 2003, p. 9).

An example of how this set of advocacies can be implemented was described by Lancaster et al. (2015), who employed the ACA competencies in their design of a university-based community center. They worked collaboratively with the community, negotiated with policy makers to secure funding, and shared information on best practices with stakeholders. Especially noteworthy, they provided trainees with concrete guidance on how to actualize social justice work in a real-world community setting.

According to Swenson (1998), as a profession, social work claims social justice as an organizing value. Drawing on Wakefield's work (1988a, 1988b), she distinguished the profession's mission as differing from medicine in its focus on "curing disease." Social work's organizing values include legal justice and having an emphasis on the "person in situation." Swenson noted that when the social worker sits with the client, social justice means

> profound appreciation for the client's strengths, contexts, and resources. . . . It means we engage in thorough analyses of professional and organizational power and actively work to increase client power relative to professionals and agencies. It means we acknowledge and articulate the client's social realities. We engage in the work of exploring our own experiences of oppression and of privilege as well. (p. 534)

Social work, too, struggles with putting the commitment into practice (Asakura & Maurer, 2018; Maschi et al., 2011). The National Association of Social Workers (NASW, 2015) encourages adherence through its competencies; social justice is considered a fundamental component of effective social work practice. NASW also identifies social justice priorities on an annual basis; examples of such are voters' rights, immigration, criminal justice/juvenile justice, economic justice, and environmental justice.

In her book *Just Practice: A Social Justice Approach to Social Work*, Finn (2020) identified the profound global and national challenges social work faces in the 21st century. They hit on all fronts: safe housing, food, water, health care, violence, war, immigration, and more. She presented a framework for social justice work that is designed to translate five key themes—meaning, context, power, history, and possibility—into concrete practice. Finn invited the reader to "take risks; to move from safe, familiar pedagogical spaces and practices; to challenge assumptions; to sit with ambiguity; and to embrace uncertainty" (p. xviii).

The competent multicultural therapist is inherently a social justice advocate. The two identities are inextricably intertwined. The charge to each maps on to the other: know your identities, respect your patient's identities, understand the political environments in which you both live, work to make them all healthier. The integration of social justice as part of the multicultural therapy curriculum has evolved in the training of future psychotherapy providers. Pedagogical applications to integrate social justice awareness, advocacy skills, and opportunities for social change action have advanced to evolve as needed extensions to the multicultural curriculum (Motulsky et al., 2014).

Any discourse on multicultural therapy must include attention to social justice. Many writers have published on this issue: Hoover (2016) on social justice and feminism; Comas-Díaz (2012b) on social justice as the next force in psychotherapy; Arczynski (2017) on social justice and group psychotherapy training; Ceballos et al. (2012) on social justice attitudes among play therapists; Pérez-Gualdrón and Yeh (2014) on counseling for social justice; and Comas-Díaz and Torres Rivera (2020) on liberation psychology, among others.

We have chosen to quote liberally from Ratts and Pedersen (2014) because their elucidation of the assumptions of social justice and the distinctions between multiculturalism and social justice bear repeating. Specifically, they asserted the following:

- There is complexity in the multiple aspects of human identity.
- Multiculturalism is broadly defined and includes all the unique dimensions that shaped human identity.

- All counseling takes place in a multicultural and sociopolitical context.
- The most important elements of multicultural and social justice competence can be learned but cannot be taught. Good teaching can, however, create the favorable conditions for multicultural and social justice competence to occur.
- Multiculturalism and social justice go hand in hand. Both are necessary conditions in any psychotherapeutic interaction.
- People experience both oppression and privilege. We are members of dominant (oppressor) and target (oppressed) groups.
- The interlocking system of power, privilege, and oppression exists on many levels and hinders human growth and development.
- Counseling that is informed by intrapsychic approaches cannot sufficiently resolve systemic based issues.
- Counseling includes both individual therapy and systems advocacy.
- Counseling can serve as a vehicle to oppress or liberate clients. (pp. x–xi)

Ratts and Pedersen (2014) described the distinction between the two philosophies of multiculturalism and social justice in terms of the focus of change. Multiculturalist perspectives focus on the individual and interpersonal dynamics. Social justice recognizes that living in an unjust system creates many of the problems the individual has to address.

> Social justice counseling addresses power dynamics, issues of equity and oppression in all of its forms. Counselors operating from a social justice perspective realize that some situations require change at the individual level and other situations call for systemic-level changes. (p. 13)

The social justice–oriented therapist needs to become an advocate for change not just within the individual but for changing the dynamics of power, equity, and oppression in the institutions and communities in which they live and work. Ratts and Pedersen ultimately proposed social justice as the fifth force in counseling given the imperative to focus on the connection between client problems and larger systemic social barriers; the personal is political, given its reliance on advocacy, given its goal of externalizing oppression, and working to connect individual counseling with system change.

How does all of this play out in the multicultural therapy room? The skeptical therapist may offer the defensive question "Am I expected to change society to help my patient?" The answer is yes. We can change society when we empower our patients by honoring their experiences of oppression and marginalization. To modify a Covey (1990) principle of "seek first to understand, then to be understood" (p. 235), the therapist should seek first to believe, then question. As noted earlier, many treatment relationships are terminated prematurely when the therapist too immediately questions the validity of the patient's experience of racism. Racism is alive and well. It is better to err (if indeed it is an error) on the side of believing the client as it has the power to nurture the therapeutic alliance. The following is an example of a client's experience.

A 55-year-old Black female patient works for a nationally known company as vice president of one of its operations. She has been working for the company for 5 years, having held several high positions in other companies. Her reviews have been stellar, and she can demonstrate that her work has positively affected the company's bottom line. She has remarked that several of her peers, who are also persons of color, have left the company in recent years. She applied for a director position and felt she did very well in the interviews. A younger White woman, who from information she uncovered did not have superior or equal credentials, was ultimately selected. She brings the issue up in treatment. What is your first thought and what would be your response or question?

While one goal of treatment may be to help the patient identify alternative ways of addressing a problem, the therapist must be cautious about offering alternative ways of perceiving the problem, particularly when racial dynamics are at play. In this example, exploring the patient's "feelings" is important but no more so than examining the realities of the racial-political environment of the workplace. Support for the patient might include assessment of pros and cons of continued employment, research on employer patterns of promotions, or even identification of legal assistance on workplace bias.

Comas-Díaz and Torres Rivera (2020) went further in suggesting that psychotherapists can successfully imitate liberation psychologists by not only respectfully receiving the patient's experiences of oppression but also by *promoting* the patient's awareness of their oppression and the structural inequalities that conspire to keep them so. Liberation psychology has a strong nexus with social justice given their parallel principles, for example, that psychological problems should be addressed by concomitantly attending to their sociopolitical etiology, depending on clients to create their own definitions of attribution and healing, and seeing problems as conflicts between individuals' experiences and their perceptions about what should be (Tate et al., 2013). A vital component of liberation psychology and social justice is understanding the etiology of oppression and its persistent pernicious effect. Recovering this awareness is critical for both the patient and the therapist. A Persian proverb says, "He who knows, and knows not that he knows, is asleep; wake him" (Anonymous; retrieved from http://www.xenodochy.org/ex/quotes/knowsnot.html). Waking the patient, educating the patient, and advocating for them ultimately become second nature to the therapist committed to social justice.

We can change society when we put our advocacy into action: attending marches, contacting legislators and governmental departments, writing editorials, visiting, volunteering, contributing money to social justice causes, and voting. We can encourage our clients and model for them social justice in action. When issues arise in the treatment room, therapists can apply a liberation psychology lens in helping them understand the oppression origins of some of their suffering and empower them to confront the system along with the symptoms. This might take many forms, including encouraging the patient to

1. study the history of their culture, particularly as it relates to intergenerational trauma;
2. explore connections between personal issues and community resources, for example, sexual abuse or grief support groups, and start one if none exist;
3. nurture or expand connections with healing practices (e.g., spiritual, communal), for example, Emotional Emancipation Circles are evidence-informed, culturally grounded self-help support groups in which Black people share stories and deepen their understanding of the impact of historical forces and their sense of self-worth;

4. monitor workplace employment practices and the workplace environment of safety;
5. serve on diversity, equity, and inclusion committees;
6. attend local government meetings to know what decisions are made and how they affect all groups (e.g., zoning decisions determine safety, economic viability, and property values);
7. participate in community action projects designed to combat systemic racism;
8. seek out groups working to eliminate racism (e.g., anti-Asian, anti-Arab, anti-Black);
9. attend Gay Pride rallies, lobby legislators to support LGBTQIA affirmative legislation, and work to establish Gay-Straight Alliance groups in schools;
10. write letters to newspaper editors and government officials regarding issues of import (e.g., minimum wage, voting rights, partnering police with mental health workers, homelessness);
11. volunteer at a food bank to combat food insecurity because studies have shown a link between volunteerism and a reduction in depressive symptoms (Creaven et al., 2018); and
12. use social media to inform and galvanize around social justice issues.

The following provide examples of client advocacy actions.

A patient of Dr. J was facing challenges in obtaining her green card. She encountered inexplicable delays and was nearing a critical point in the process. She was anxious and moderately depressed and could focus on little else in the session. The therapist knew someone who worked in the U.S. Citizenship and Immigration Services office. She conferred with him, and he agreed to meet with the patient to explore the delays. He was ultimately able to expedite the process.

Another patient, a 22-year-old, faced prison time for speeding and fleeing the police while carrying a weapon. He had left a meeting with friends where he'd said goodbye before planning to kill himself. There were many other issues at play that gave rise to the suicide attempt (loss of a significant relationship, failure to gain admission to a desired program, financial and familial stress, theft charge); these were being addressed in therapy. Though his depression remitted during treatment, he still faced prison time. The therapist was asked and agreed to write letters on his behalf to the prosecutor. It would be great to say the story had a happily-ever-after ending and he did not have to serve time; nonetheless, the therapeutic material did mitigate the sentencing. More important, the patient experienced his therapist's active commitment to "his" social justice. As the therapist, Dr. J can report that the patient is now married and has built a successful engineering career.

We can change society when we work on health care, economic and educational reform, ensure that our offices and meeting places are barrier free, lobby for LGBTQ equality, fight against racist immigration practices, and support freedom for and from religion. The multicultural therapist can advocate for social justice, as the saying goes, by "speaking truth to power" and privilege.

Psychologists have seized opportunities to serve social justice causes at the highest level of discourse. For example, APA is often called on to submit amicus briefs in cases brought before the U.S. Supreme Court. In these cases, psychologists do not actually give testimony but provide scientific expertise that informs these briefs. Our scientific expertise has been used to address a wide range of social justice issues including abortion, affirmative action, battered women's syndrome, child abuse and child sexual abuse, civil commitment, competency, death penalty, disabilities rights under the Americans With Disabilities Act (ADA), duty to warn and protect, eyewitness identification research, gender identity, false confessions, juvenile sentencing, medication (right to refuse), rights of incarcerated persons to mental health treatment, sexual harassment, and sexual orientation, among others (APA, n.d.). In one case in 2019, Dr. Francisco Sánchez provided input into the amicus brief that APA filed with the U.S. Supreme Court (Brief of Amicus Curiae American Psychological Association et al., 2020) on behalf of LGBTQ+ employees claiming workplace discrimination. The employees in several cases had been terminated because their employers believed they failed to "conform with expected sexual stereotypes based on their birth gender." Testimony cited scientific data showing that workplace discrimination against sexual and gender minorities is not only illegal (per Title VII of the Civil Rights Act of 1964) but is also "associated with negative outcomes in psychological and physiological health. Sexual and gender minorities who experience discrimination in the workplace may also experience minority stress-related psychological distress and illness, substance use and even physical violence" (p. 23). Fortunately, the Supreme Court of the United States (SCOTUS) released a ruling on June 15, 2020, that protected LGBTQ people from work discrimination (Sherman, 2020). The SCOTUS determined that the landmark Civil Rights Act does indeed forbid an employer from treating a person who is gay or transgender for traits or actions it would not have questioned in others. The contribution of psychologists' expertise in cases such as this goes a long way in promoting the mental health of members of society. There seems to be an understanding that the quest to transform this country cannot be limited to challenging its brutal police alone (K.-Y. Taylor, 2020); legislative and community advocacy are necessary. People are also rightly demanding to be free of the coercion of poverty and inequality. K.-Y. Taylor (2020), author of the 2019 *Race for Profit: How Banks and the Real Estate Industry Undermined Black Home-ownership*, reminded us of other historical demonstrations and protests against police abuse. She also warned us that in the 1990s the response was a convergence of the political right and the Democratic party to engage in harsh budget cuts of social programs, including food stamps. The effects have continued to this day. Also, in the 1990s when a new crime bill was introduced that added thousands more police to the streets, the Democratic party had a new emphasis on law and order, with expanded policing, prisons, and death sentences. Taylor warned that the current criminal justice system and the absence of a welfare state have contributed to inequality. Our social justice advocacy must deal with economic stagnation in African American communities, residential segregation, job discrimination, underresourced public schools, and disparities in health care, among others, by making space for new politics, new ideas, new formations, and new people.

As noted in Chapter 3, the video released of police officer Derek Chauvin's horrific killing of an African American man, George Floyd, in Minneapolis in late May 2020 brought into the public's unavoidable awareness the concept of "dying while Black." In the same week a White woman, Amy Cooper, in Central Park, New York, tried to weaponize her Whiteness by calling the police on Christian Cooper, an African American birdwatcher, who had asked her to leash her dog. She weaponized her White privilege to intimidate a Black man, knowing the symbolic threat. Other deaths by police brutality in the same period included Breonna Taylor, killed in her bed while she slept when three plain-clothes officers barged into the wrong house searching for someone who had already been arrested, as well as Ahmaud Arbery, killed while jogging by White neighbors who falsely claimed he was guilty of robbery and took it upon themselves to be judge, jury, and executioners in the exercise of their racism.

An international monumental outcry of protests, mostly peaceful, continued for months across the country, and even internationally. The sheer scale of the uprisings of multiracial crowds in cities large and small has been surprising. Two weeks after the brutal murder of George Floyd, more than 17,000 National Guard troops had been deployed, more than 10,000 people arrested, more than 12 people killed, and curfews imposed in at least 30 cities (K.-Y. Taylor, 2020). Solidarity demonstrations were organized in international cities such as Dublin, Paris, Berlin, London, Accra, and more. Through protest, people are demonstrating their understanding of how racist attitudes are pervasive and institutionalized. Diverse members of society have stood in solidarity with the antiracist Black Lives Matter movement.

Concurrent with the sociopolitical changes was the worldwide COVID-19 epidemic. Compared with White Americans, a disproportionate number of Black, Indigenous, People of Color (BIPOC) have been affected by the pandemic (Centers for Disease Control [CDC], 2020a, 2020b, 2020c; Cordes & Castro, 2020; Millett et al., 2020; Novacek et al., 2020), and their overrepresentation in jobs that are considered essential, their dependence on public transportation, closer living quarters, barriers to access to health care, among other factors, have increased this disparity. Perpetuating the imbalance is the report from the National Academy of Sciences (Andrasfay & Goldman, 2021) projecting that COVID-19 will reduce the life expectancy of Black and Latinx populations 3 to 4 times that for White people. This context has likely contributed to the unbearable pain and concern about a long history of an aggressive, brutal, and abusive police culture against people of color.

In the United States, many groups, organizations, and corporate companies expressed concern about the blatant aggression by police as well as about the racism that underlies it. *The Wall Street Journal* (Pacheco & Stamm, 2020) provided an analysis of what 35 executives of big companies said in their public comments about the killing of George Floyd. Most companies condemned racism and called for unity. Even the NFL commissioner, Roger Goodell, finally admitted the league has been at fault for not listening to its players denouncing racism:

> We, the NFL, condemn racism and the systematic oppression of Black People. We, the NFL, admit we were wrong for not listening to NFL players earlier and encourage all to speak out and peacefully protest. We, the NFL, believe Black Lives Matter. (Goodell, 2020)

The American Psychiatric Association in 2021 issued an *Apology to Black, Indigenous and People of Color for Its Support of Structural Racism in Psychiatry*. They admitted that their psychiatric practices limited quality access to psychiatric care, victimized BIPOC through experimentation, racialized diagnoses, propagated dangerous stereotypes, and fundamentally "contributed to perpetuation of structural racism that has adversely impacted not just its own BIPOC members, but also psychiatric patients across America" (para. 2). They pledged to work to achieve social equality, health equality and fairness that all human beings deserve.

There are some hopeful signs on the horizon. Several jurisdictions, including New York City; Eugene, Oregon; Seattle, Washington; and Albuquerque, New Mexico, have adopted policies that recognize the need for more informed police interventions (Butler & Sheriff, 2020). Police departments are partnering with mental health agencies to include mental health and crisis professionals as responders to mental health calls. The lack of police mental health training too often has led to disastrous results including fatalities. When lack of training is combined with health disparities, communities of color are disproportionately affected. It is an optimistic though reasonable inference that as more mental health professionals are multiculturally competent, those skills will manifest, adding to the effectiveness of these programs.

It is indeed hopeful that the Black Lives Matter movement, fueled by several tragic deaths and built upon a history of political and racial dissent, has gathered a strength not seen before. We hope that the protests propelled by these killings lead to substantive changes not only in the aggressive and militaristic police culture but also in the institutionalized and ingrained racism in this country. The social justice possibilities are virtually unlimited. Psychologists have the science, knowledge, and abilities to advocate for change through the conversations we can have in the therapy room, classroom, living room, conference room, and community room, through amici briefs and taking to the streets.

6

Multiculturalism in Education, Training, and Professional Development

A s predicted nearly 2 decades ago (Norcross et al., 2002), multi-cultural therapy has been a growing force in the discipline and practice of psychology. As we noted earlier, scholars and practitioners alike have embraced multicultural perspectives as central to their theories and research.

The incorporation of multicultural principles and practices into education and training aids the development of multicultural competence; therefore, in this chapter, we look at the ways education and training guidelines, licensing requirements, and continuing education have recognized and incorporated multiculturalism and diversity principles throughout the educational and practice lifespan in psychology and other allied disciplines. They are summarized here not only to highlight the growth, expansion, and acceptance of multiculturalism into mental health fields but also to facilitate awareness of the rules of development and

https://doi.org/10.1037/0000279-006
Multicultural Therapy: A Practice Imperative, by M. J. T. Vasquez and J. D. Johnson
Copyright © 2022 by the American Psychological Association. All rights reserved.

maintenance of multicultural skills and competencies. Trainees and practitioners are also encouraged to be vigilant in monitoring programs' fidelity to the multicultural principles as a professional and ethical responsibility. Some clinical application issues are explored, along with other disciplines such as counseling and social work, and Canadian guidelines are also cited. We provide examples of multiculturalism's application in supervision and research as well as within couples, family, group, and play therapies.

PEDAGOGY

The methods and practices of teaching multicultural psychology are described briefly here in a developmental sequence. Curricula at the high school, undergraduate, master's graduate, and doctoral graduate education levels are described, and the teaching of multicultural curriculum issues in counseling, social work, assessment, and research is also discussed. Teaching of multicultural therapy in clinical supervision is addressed.

High School

Beginning at the high school level, standards for psychology curricula include an overarching theme that addresses "a multicultural and global perspective that recognizes how diversity is important to understanding psychology" (American Psychological Association [APA], 2011b, p. 2). As noted in earlier chapters of this monograph, the "psychology" of a person or group is context dependent; therefore, high school psychology teachers are advised that they should incorporate diversity issues throughout their courses and point out the limitations of the generalizability of Western scholarship to a global community (APA, 2011b). Thus, high school psychology teachers should encourage critical thinking about worldviews and include instruction on intersectionality.

Cokley (2021) suggested that critics of critical race theory and its instruction use it to falsely decry any examination of systemic racism as "anti-American" and offered, instead, that teaching critical race theory is patriotic. He reminded us that critical race theory posits that racism is not simply acts of individual bias or prejudice; it is embedded in institutions, policies, and legal systems, and as such systemic racism is still a part of U.S. society. Far from perfect, the United States remains a work in progress. Although discussions about race in the classroom are difficult, they need not be oppressive or guilt-inducing and can contribute to improving society.

Also practicing within the educational environment, school psychologists wield tremendous influence over the lives of their students. Testing, classroom placement decisions, discipline, and designation for special education programs have profound effects on students' futures, particularly those of Black, Indigenous, People of Color (BIPOC) students (Anyon et al., 2018; Frey, 2019; Grindal et al., 2019). In recognition of the historically disparate treatment of BIPOC students in K–12 education, school psychologists are enjoined by their certifying body, the National Association of School Psychologists (2020), to "recognize that equitable practices for diverse student populations, respect for diversity in development and learning, and advocacy for social justice are foundational to effective service delivery" (p. 8).

Undergraduate Education

The California State University Board of Trustees took a major step in July 2020 when it voted to require inclusion of a course addressing ethnic studies and social justice in its general education requirements (California State University, 2020). It was the first substantial change to the general education requirements in the university system in 40 years. The potential impact is significant; California State University is the largest 4-year higher education system in the country, educating 482,000 students annually. While a single course is insufficient to develop multicultural competence, instituting such a requirement may encourage other universities to take similar steps toward providing a foundation for students in every major to apply a global awareness and social justice lens to their studies and future lives and work. Infusing diversity and social justice concepts throughout the undergraduate learning process provides a minimum level of awareness and knowledge to instill a real appreciation of diversity concerns.

While the addition of an ethnic studies and social justice course may facilitate the goals of undergraduate psychology education, the commitment to diversity training in psychology undergraduate majors, specifically, goes further "by ensuring that diversity is *not just a stand-alone experience but a central feature* [emphasis added] of all student learning goals" (APA, 2013, p. 13). The *APA Guidelines for the Undergraduate Psychology Major: Version 2.0* propose that "diversity not only be incorporated in one of the five domains of effort in *Guidelines 2.0* but that diversity issues need to be recognized as an essential feature and commitment of each of the five domains" (APA, 2013, p. 12). Seizing the opportunity to nurture critical thinking the instructor must commit to ensuring that multicultural and social justice concepts are central in all psychology courses taught. Meyers (2007) recommended that this might be accomplished practically through themes (e.g., explaining that psychology is not always value free, encouraging students to speak out for change in social action projects, promote students' self-examination during in-class time) to help students appreciate how the pairing of psychological knowledge with social justice helps them become engaged, informed global citizens.

Master's Education

Beyond the general awareness and knowledge of diversity and social justice that high school and undergraduates are expected to master, graduate students are expected to build upon that foundation and develop skills to competently work with diverse groups and communities (APA, 2018c). Such competence includes a cultural humility orientation "characterized by respect and lack of superiority toward an individual's cultural background and experience" (Hook et al., 2015, p. 1) in assessing the impact of differing backgrounds and worldviews. It is difficult to overestimate the value of impressing on therapists, early in training, the importance of approaching the treatment relationship with an attitude of openness versus superiority. Beginning and seasoned therapists should be familiar with the research that shows that cultural humility facilitates positive treatment outcomes as it is associated with stronger relationship bonds (Davis et al., 2013) and helps the therapist learn from the client in an interested and respectful manner (Hook et al., 2013).

Doctoral Education

Doctoral programs that provide training in clinical psychology, counseling psychology, school psychology, and other areas of practice are reviewed by APA's Commission on Accreditation (CoA). CoA holds that "programs that are accredited to provide training in health service psychology prepare individuals to work in diverse settings with diverse populations" (APA, 2015b, p. 2). CoA identifies individual and cultural diversity as a competency relevant to advanced practice. It also assesses a program's systematic and sustained effort to attract residents and staff from diverse backgrounds.

The following vignette is an example of an academic institution's failure when it pays lip service to equity, diversity, and inclusion goals in education and training but does not follow through with the necessary resources for training the next generation of mental health providers. Having already earned a master's degree in school psychology, Chavonne was admitted into a clinical doctoral program at a nationally recognized university in the Midwest. She knew the program's history of "letting Blacks in but not letting them out." She persevered, completing all of the coursework with good to excellent grades. She chose a dissertation topic with a culturally specific focus. Despite multiple revisions, corrections, and reworking, the proposal was never "acceptable" to her committee. Ultimately, she "timed out" and reached the limit of time allotted to complete a dissertation. She still does not have a doctorate and has given up the dream. She knew there were clear barriers to her success: a lack of faculty mentors of color, a culturally insensitive and perhaps even culturally hostile thesis advisor, and a failure on the university's part to create a multiculturally supportive environment overall.

From a clinical perspective, if you encountered Chavonne in the therapy office, how would you conceptualize her experience in the context of social justice? Should you feel any obligation to advocate for increased diversity in staffing at the university? Should you bring up or acknowledge racism as a part of the dialogue, and if so, how? As noted in Chapter 5, favoring the therapeutic alliance, and in the spirit of believing our clients, the clinician should avoid immediately challenging or questioning the patient's perception of racism. T. B. Smith and Trimble (2016) noted that meta-analytic research data show that therapists better assist clients by framing discussions of race in terms of resilience and resistance (p. 179). N. L. Phillips et al. (2015) also noted that the conventional therapeutic approach to experiences of racial oppression is to emphasize coping, self-efficacy, or adaptation. A focus on resilience and resistance allows the client to find her own strengths from identifying coping skills that help her reduce her stress response to disrupting systemic racism within her institution. Identifying and facilitating the development of resilience and resistance to oppression coincide with multicultural and liberation psychology approaches.

Discussion of the foregoing guidelines and competencies raises questions about how courses focusing on competencies should be structured. Should they be offered as single courses, multiple courses to be taken in conjunction with any training orientation, or a combination of both? While there is faint support for offering a single course, there may be some value in requiring at least minimal exposure to all students (as in California). Even one course has the potential to instill some appreciation of the importance of culture and the value of diversity.

According to Mio (2003), however, a single course is insufficient for competent psychotherapeutic practice and cannot prepare trainees to treat culturally diverse clients. He recommended an integrative model, a cluster of courses that cover "assimilation/acculturation, intelligence testing, White privilege, racism, emic–etic distinctions, individualism–collectivism distinctions, research and methodological issues, racial identity, and norms, values, and other issues related to specific groups of diversity" (e.g., women, gays and lesbians, individuals with disabilities, and older adults; p. 135). Michael and Bartoli (2017) agreed that the one course model is not preferred but also said that "multiple courses" would be taxing on a program's credits. Even the "inclusion" model, they noted, suffers from difficulties in guaranteeing uniformity of materials across courses. They have designed a model that combines the one course with the infusion approach. It is enhanced by the inclusion of multicultural self-awareness labs that raise students' consciousness about the role they play in clinical work. Clearly, the options are more extensive than viewing it either as a stand-alone approach or infusion into all courses.

T. B. Smith and Trimble (2016) described multicultural psychology as "a construction project, not a single edifice but a vast complex of buildings. In a word, it is a community, a community in which all are welcomed, none excluded" (p. 246). Regardless of the level of offerings, the challenge is to keep the construction going by offering relevant courses wherever possible by teaching a single course, multiple courses, attending to cultural diversity in all psychology courses, or offering a comprehensive multicultural curriculum. With an increasingly diverse student population and awareness of global sensibilities, it is important to teach appreciation of the central role and relevance of culture. The challenge/opportunity is to keep the community open to all, including engineers, lawyers, accountants, teachers, and culinary artists, by infusing multiculturalism into all course offerings. Aragón et al. (2017) evaluated two approaches to increasing diversity in college-level STEM (science, technology, engineering, mathematics) classes and found that a color-blind approach, or downplaying differences, was less effective in generating inclusive teaching practices than a multicultural approach of embracing differences. They found that a multicultural approach facilitates underrepresented students' sense of belonging.

Counseling and Related Educational Programs

In the field of counseling, educational master's and doctoral degree programs are accredited by the Council for Accreditation of Counseling and Related Educational Programs (CACREP). Its standards for all entry-level and doctoral-level programs require competencies in social and cultural diversity. Among others, these include multicultural counseling competencies, cultural identity development, social justice and advocacy, bidirectional effects of power and privilege for counselors and clients, impact of heritage, acculturation, and beliefs in shaping worldviews (CACREP, 2016). The American Counseling Association (ACA, 2015) developed multicultural and social justice counseling competencies to prepare both privileged and marginalized counselors in the four domains of self-awareness, client worldview, counseling relationship, and counselor and advocacy interventions. They embedded D. W. Sue et al.'s (1992) model of attitudes and beliefs, knowledge, skills, and action competencies. The interweaving of counseling and advocacy highlights the recognition within the field of counseling of the fundamental importance of social justice to the definition of competent practice.

Social Work

The ethical codes for cultural competence in the field of social work (Council on Social Work Education, 2015) provide a thorough set of standards that include Standard 9: Language and Communication:

> Social workers shall provide and advocate for effective communication with clients of all cultural groups, including people of limited English proficiency or low literacy skills, people who are blind or have low vision, people who are deaf or hard of hearing, and people with disabilities. (Goode & Jones, 2009, p. 5)

Their terminology calls out cultural humility, intersectionality, and "cissexism" (discrimination against transgender individuals). For each of the 10 standards, the National Association of Social Workers provides an interpretation and a list of indicators; it is a comprehensive resource not only for social work trainees and practicing professionals but for practitioners in other disciplines as well.

Multicultural Training in Assessment

Training multiculturally competent evaluators who are knowledgeable of the limitations of assessment practices, from intake procedures to standardized assessment instruments, is critical not only to the science and practice of psychology but also to the individuals and communities affected (Constantine, 1998; de las Fuentes et al., 2013). Consider the harm that has resulted from a long history of placing children from particular ethnic groups into inferior education programs and special education programs on the basis of biased or unfair assessments and assessment practices. For example, in the mid-1930s, Sánchez (1934) criticized studies on IQ in Mexican and Spanish-speaking children for their failure to consider many linguistic, social, environmental, and cultural factors. These biased studies informed policies justifying school segregation and inferior educational resources and opportunities for children in the southwest United States for decades. Nearly 40 years later, in *Diana v. State Board of Education* (1970), the problems were still being litigated. This case found that California schools were labeling Mexican American children as "mentally retarded" on the basis of a single IQ test conducted in the student's nonnative language. The ruling set the precedent that testing should be nonverbal or conducted in the student's native language.

Larry P. v. Riles (1979) was a California class-action case focused on the biased testing of African American children that argued that those children had been inappropriately placed in "educable mental retardation" (EMR) classrooms solely on the basis of an IQ score. At the time, 25% of the population enrolled in EMR classes were Black children, but they were only 10% of the general student population. The court ruled that the test contained racial and cultural biases, discriminated against racial minorities, and was designed and standardized on the basis of an all-White population. As a result, the court ordered that IQ tests could not be used as the sole basis for placing children into special education, a ruling that was later overturned. California may now conduct intelligence tests only if they have been proven reliable and have been normed on representative populations.

The APA (2017a) *Ethical Principles of Psychologists and Code of Conduct* (APA Ethics Code) urges psychologists to "use assessment instruments whose validity and reliability have been established for use with members of the population tested. When such validity or reliability has not been established, psychologists describe the strengths and limitations of test results and interpretation" (p. 13). In addition, evaluators are urged to attend to the issue of an individual's *language preference*, identifying concerns regarding translation of instruments and norm groups. Cultural factors relevant in the assessment process include relevant generational history (e.g., number of generations in the country, manner of coming to the country); citizenship or residency status; fluency in "standard" English or other language; availability of family support and community resources; level of education and reading level; change in social status as a result of coming to this country (for immigrant or refugee); work history, and level of stress related to acculturation and/or oppression (APA, 2003, 2017a).

Effective psychotherapy invariably involves clinical diagnosis and assessment. Leong et al. (2020) pointed out that optimal interventions are derived from accurate diagnoses but warned that there are threats to the cultural validity (efficiency of a clinical diagnosis in considering the import of critical cultural factors) of diagnoses. For example, the presumption of psychological uniformity of symptoms and course regardless of culture or ethnicity or using a general group versus a within group perspective can lead to misdiagnoses. Leong and Kalibatseva (2016) identified therapist bias as a threat to the cultural validity of clinical diagnosis. Prejudice, ignorance, and culture-based countertransference are illustrative of therapist bias. In a 2018 survey of its members, the Canadian Psychiatric Association reported that 79% reported discriminating toward a BIPOC patient. Further, 53% of them observed other professionals in the medical field discriminate against a psychiatry patient (Canadian Mental Health Association, 2018).

De las Fuentes et al. (2013) addressed unique issues related to forensic evaluations of immigrant women, and S. R. Smith and Krishnamurthy's (2018) edited contribution, "Diversity-Sensitive Personality Assessment," provided a comprehensive update to address how traditional approaches to psychological assessment contain assumptions that may be inappropriate or possibly antagonistic to many culturally or demographically diverse groups. They conveyed the complex ways in which individuals' personal characteristics, backgrounds, and viewpoints intersect and pointed out that the field of emotion expression suggests that individuals from different cultures display and experience emotions based on the "rules" taught by the culture with which they most identify. Being open to and respectful of "rule sets" from our own cultural contexts reduces chances of misinterpreting patients' behaviors. These authors reminded us that an assessment is a snapshot, and the full appraisal of the fluid, ongoing process of development may not be captured if the context isn't considered. They also suggested strategies for selection of instruments, including culturally specific instruments, and encouraged us to ask, "What is the theory behind the instrument? What is the sample make-up and size?" Many important considerations in report writing, ethics, supervision and training, and research are addressed as well.

Diversity Issues in Training Researchers

Myths persist about the lack of "place" for culture in psychological research despite fair consensus around the belief that "all human behavior is culturally informed" (Kagawa-Singer et al., 2015). The failure to consider culture may be due to the lack of an agreed-on definition (Kagawa-Singer et al., 2015), that it is simply ignored as a trait that does not impact generalizability (S. Sue, 1999), or a belief that culture is irrelevant to basic psychological processes (Chiao et al., 2013; Sternberg, 2014; C. Taylor et al., 2013). The data that flow from research that fails to consider culture have extraordinary power and lasting impact in that they not only undergird education and practice but also influence worldviews (S. Sue, 1999).

Hall et al. (2016) highlighted the importance of attending to ethnocultural diversity in research describing and identifying strengths and weaknesses of three broad research perspectives (generalizability research: seeking universalities; group difference research: exploring the limits of generalizability; and multicultural psychology research: measuring within-cultural group perspectives without comparison to another group). They proposed a fourth perspective, ethnocultural research, that incorporates the perspectives of members of ethnocultural communities while deemphasizing generalizability. It goes beyond simple inclusion and post hoc inferences about differences to "conceptual models that guide the selection of participants, research questions, manipulations, measures, analyses, and data interpretation" (Hall et al., 2016, p. 46).

Hall et al. (2016) and others have pointed to the importance of increasing the presence and visibility of underrepresented groups in psychological research. Despite the National Institutes of Health's (NIH's) requirement that grantees demonstrate analysis of clinical trials variables on minorities and women (NIH, 2001, 2018), minority research continues to lag. Wang (2016) reported that 96% of participant samples in psychological research come from Western, educated, industrialized, rich, and democratic (WEIRD) societies yet these societies constitute only 16% of the world's population. Medin and Lee (2012) suggested that validity discussions in the sciences must include more than controls and replicability but must also consider choices about what problems and populations to study and procedures and measures to be used. They pointed to the strong correlation between social science researchers and the people they study: White, middle-class researchers largely study White, middle-class populations.

Expanding cultural variation in research populations increases the generalizability of findings, reducing the need for further verification. Wang (2016) cited research that supports the contention that culture is relevant to processes typically considered to be basic, that is, outside cultural influences such as sensation, face processing, color perception, even taste preferences. Persons from cultures that prioritize collectivist over individualist orientations also tend to focus less on self-goals rather than group goals. This impacts the focus, precision, and salience of recollections prompted in therapy. There are significant long-term effects of cultural differences, as Wang noted. For example, in a longitudinal study of European American and Chinese immigrant children in the United States, Wang (2008) found that European American children with higher levels of emotional knowledge were more socially competent and exhibited fewer internalizing problems. Chinese children with such skills, on the other hand, were more likely to have social adjustment problems. She found this to be so when children were assessed at age 3.5 and again at age 7, demonstrating that while emotional intelligence may be highly regarded in Western cultures, it may be an interpersonal liability in others. Findings such as these may have significant relevance to multicultural therapy as they highlight the value and need for further inquiry on research assumptions about the relevance of culture.

Paquin et al. (2019) identified a number of concerns that should be addressed in the conduct of ethical and socially just research. They pointed out the fallacy of the notion of incompatibility between social justice and scientific inquiry in psychotherapy research and further examined the challenges of adhering to some of the APA (2017a) Ethics Code, for example, nonmaleficence (do no harm), by ensuring that research does not contribute to systematic oppression, and beneficence (aim to help), which must be considered in the choice of research design. For example, randomized controlled trials (RCTs) are generally considered the gold standard of psychological research for determining causality and treatment effectiveness; however, they do not always function de facto as "the" legitimate design, particularly for research with ethnic minorities. Despite the NIH's (2001) mandate for increased inclusion of women and minorities as subjects, there have not been significant increases (Geller et al., 2018). There are a number of problems associated with the inclusion or exclusion of participants from diverse backgrounds in RCTs. First, too few studies actually described characteristics of the samples employed; too few of the ones that did have the characteristics listed have sufficient diverse representation upon which to report findings (Polo et al., 2019; Williams et al., 2010). This scarcity calls into question the generalizability of research findings (Williams et al., 2010). RCTs stand as the fulcrum on which evidence is balanced. Aisenberg (2008) identified five factors contributing to the exclusion of people of color in research on evidence-based practices (EBPs), asserting that it

> (a) prevents strong and clear conclusions about the efficacy of most mental health EBPs with regard to people of color, (b) raises serious questions about the legitimacy of disseminating EBPs to ethnic populations, especially because most EBPs have been developed without consideration of the cultural context and identity of communities of color, (c) helps promote the use of standardized measures not normed for diverse ethnic groups, (d) scant research examines the heterogeneity within ethnic groups, including ethnic differences in

patterns of mental disorders and treatment outcomes, and (e) the lack of representative numbers of ethnic minority populations in RCTs thwarts the attainment of a primary objective of EBP, namely, the distribution of treatment to address disparities. (pp. 95–96)

Still, there are other factors affecting research that are more personally salient to the history of Black people in the United States. Resistance to participating in institutional studies of various kinds owes some of its beginnings to the Tuskegee syphilis study (Centers for Disease Control and Prevention, 2021). As the details are readily available in the public domain, only a brief summary is presented here. For 40 years, from 1932 to 1972, the U.S. Public Health Service solicited 600 poor Black men to participate in a study promising free medical care. Instead, they studied the impact of untreated syphilis in the 399 men who had the disease. They did not inform the men of their diagnoses, nor did they provide any medical treatment as promised (even after penicillin became available in 1947). These men developed severe disease at the hands of health service providers and public health researchers that could have been prevented. Distrust of "the system" persists and has *some* impact on Black people's hesitancy in the COVID-19 vaccination programs. *Some* is emphasized because, as Bajaj and Stanford (2021) stated,

These historical traumas certainly provide critical context for interpreting present-day occurrences. But attributing distrust primarily to these instances ignores the everyday racism that Black communities face. Every day, Black Americans have their pain denied, their conditions misdiagnosed, and necessary treatment withheld by physicians. (p. 1)

The key element in RCTs, random assignment to treatment conditions, may pose problems for ethnic minorities. Just as Tuskegee lifts the specter of inclusion, randomized assignment to the "no treatment" group may raise concerns about not receiving needed care (Corrigan & Salzer, 2003; Lau et al., 2010). There may be suspicions that assignments are based on factors other than randomness. There always exists for the researcher the ethical dilemma of determining what to do if the treatment is deemed effective before the study ends.

Other research methodologies (e.g., qualitative research) can be used to describe the subjective lived experience of people; for example, "public health and ethnographic research are especially useful for tracking the availability, utilization, and acceptance of mental health treatments as well as suggesting ways of altering these treatments to maximize their utility in a given social context" (APA Presidential Task Force on Evidence-Based Practice, 2006, p. 274). Hughes and DuMont (2002) reported that the use of focus groups in their study of dual-career African American families' experience of discrimination allowed direct observation of groups' points of commonality and convergence but also led to the elucidation of unknown issues the researchers had not considered and led to the development of additional assessment items.

Wang's (2016) insistence that all researchers become cultural psychologists, by seeing the advantages that cultural differences might bring to their work, highlighted opportunities for collaboration between the practice and research communities. Data derived from these collaborations should yield the most reliable, valid, and generalizable results. Direct collaboration may not be possible, however, and in these instances (though not in these instances alone), the cultural representativeness of peer research reviewers should be explored. Paquin et al. (2019) also urged research psychologists to "actively assume social and personal responsibility for how, what, and why we engage in psychotherapy science" (p. 499).

In the consideration of a number of research dilemmas, Owen (2013) suggested that researchers do a better job of capturing the intersectionality of multiple identities in cultural process psychotherapy research, such as assessing clients' multicultural identities via open-ended questions and assessing the saliency of these identities. He also recommended that, with advances in technology, we may be able to do a better job in coding and capturing the complex interactions between facets thought to be more relational (e.g., alliance, empathy) and the more technique related aspects (e.g., challenges, interpretations) of psychotherapy. These are not stand-alone processes, and a psychotherapist makes moment-by-moment decisions as to which interventions to engage. Capturing the unique aspects of the interactions would help advance our understanding of how best to approach interventions.

Richeson's (2018) research focused on demographic changes within the United States, explaining why diversity efforts fail (Michel, 2018). She identified a concept called the diversity paradox. It is a belief that if an outgroup's status increases, it will threaten to usurp the status and position of influence of the ingroup. Hofstra et al. (2020) examined whether the concept related also to scientists. They followed the careers of a large number of doctoral recipients in the United States, looking at their career attainments, scientific innovations, and rewards for their innovations, and found that despite gender and racial minorities in the study producing higher rates of scientific novelty, their offerings were devalued and discounted. One might conclude that even though diversity makes better science, it also breeds contempt. Ultimately, the value of diversity in research is being beyond the clear equity advantages to scientists, by enhancing the knowledge base of psychological science and practice. As Medin and Lee (2012) reported, "diversity makes better science" via the diversity of ideas, methods, populations, practitioners, problems, and practice sites.

Clinical Supervision

Clinical supervision, as defined by of number of experts in the field, is "provided by a more senior professional to one in a more junior position, for enhancing professional functioning, monitoring the quality of professional services, and serving as a gatekeeper for the profession" (Milne & Watkins, 2014, p. 3; see also Bernard & Goodyear, 2014; Falender et al., 2014). Multicultural supervision attends to culture and diversity issues as a core component of supervision (Hook, Watkins, et al., 2016). The scholarship on clinical supervision has increasingly acknowledged the importance and impact of multicultural perspectives on the development of the emerging therapist, the client, and the supervisor (Hook, Watkins, et al., 2016; Peters, 2017; J. C. Phillips et al., 2017; Porter, 1995). While some training programs have yet to infuse multicultural competence throughout their training offerings, clinical supervision provides an opportunity to augment the training by honing clinical skills and facilitating the bidirectional growth of the supervisor and trainee, to the ultimate benefit of the client. Falender and Shafranske (2016) suggested that clinical supervision is dynamic and always developing, even for the seasoned professional.

Multicultural therapy perspectives in supervision challenge the supervisor to attend to metacompetence, "reflection on what we do not know, which involves the ongoing self-assessment of capabilities and limitations" (Falender & Shafranske, 2016, p. 8), is open to multilayered feedback, and presses for maintenance of competence.

The *APA Guidelines for Clinical Supervision in Health Service Psychology* (APA, 2014a) addresses multicultural issues and declares that diversity competence is an inseparable and essential component of supervision competence. The guidelines emphasize the importance of self-awareness, ongoing plans for enhancement of diversity competence, ongoing training, knowledge about the effects of bias, prejudice and stereotyping, and familiarity with the scholarly literature concerning diversity competence in supervision.

Clinical supervision provides another layer of opportunity for the supervisee to receive training and guidance in developing culturally oriented practice skills. This is expressly important if the supervisee's training program failed to prepare its students to work in a culturally diverse world. Here, again, the value of cultural humility is elevated if the supervisor is also at a nascent stage of competence. The culturally humble supervisor avoids the trap of false bravado and embraces an attitude of a joint journey of discovery. Even culturally experienced supervisors model cultural humility in their willingness to learn from and about the supervisee, who may or may not be overtly similar to the supervisor.

Falender et al. (2014) focused on the importance of attitude in the supervisory relationship. They noted that the knowledge and skills components of cultural competence are well addressed in multicultural supervision literature, but attitudes received much less focus. They posited that attention to supervisees' attitudes and values may indeed be the essential element in aiding supervisee multicultural competence development.

Hook et al. (2015) described several approaches the supervisor can take to facilitate supervisees' progress toward cultural humility. They encouraged supervisor assessment of and feedback on strengths and weakness; supervisee self-evaluation, for example, exploration of family of origin beliefs, attitudes, and values; and observation of clinical work, noting use of open-ended questions or avoidance of cultural issues.

An example is offered here that combines Falender et al.'s (2014) elevation of attitude and Hook et al.'s (2015) encouragement of feedback. While it is considered a part of the supervisor's role to provide feedback to the supervisee, in this case the supervisee provided feedback on the supervisor's attitude. The pair consisted of Dr. J and a clinician with whom she had had a supervisory relationship that ultimately became a consultation relationship for more than 15 years, continuing to date. The supervisee, a White female, felt a combination of freedom and fret in bringing up race-related issues with the Black female supervisor. She noted that as an early-career practitioner she felt that the tone of the relationship welcomed discussion about racial issues, but the power dynamic sometimes discouraged disagreement. By way of example, she noted that she disagreed with the supervisor about whether race needed to be identified on written evaluations. The supervisor had noted that biases sometimes accrue to race and ethnicity, even presumed from certain ethnically associated names. The clinician believed even at the time that reports were incomplete without identifying race, noting an occasion when the supervisor made an incorrect assumption about the race of a White person based on name. She acceded at the time, believing that the supervisor was insistent on excluding race. As her training ended and her career progressed, she made the considered decision to include race in her reports. In later consultation she revealed her early dilemma and ultimate resolution. Supervision is not about imposing a value system but exposing and inviting examination of the values and beliefs of both parties.

In later consultations, the clinician provided feedback to the supervisor about her openness to discuss contemporary race-related issues not necessarily pertaining to therapy cases. She recalled occasions where the supervisor shut down discussion in a way that she felt was dismissive and recalled occasions she felt the supervisor's input was instructive, and she was challenged to examine her attitudes. Recent consultations have been experienced as a safe place to question, to "check her assumptions," a phrase used by a workplace supervisor that was perceived as critical.

The clinician's overall feedback indicated that the supervisor's open and direct style allowed her to feel comfortable in "asking." That style served as a model that she could observe and draw from as she developed her own style—that lead to growth. She specifically noted that supervisor's frank approach taught her to be more direct and less worried about being misunderstood. She stated, "Misunderstandings and hurts happen in human interaction. In my view, being open to listen, consider, alter opinion based on new information, and forgive misunderstandings goes a long way in the supervisor/supervisee relationship" (personal communication, June 18, 2021).

The supervisor's assessment of the clinician's attitude included an openness to input, a willingness to "try on" the supervisor's perspective even though she did not agree. The impact of the power differential is a mainstay in supervision and should always be under consideration. From the supervisor's perspective, multicultural supervision should allow the clinician significant leeway to follow their own leanings (barring any untoward effects on the patient); it leads to authentic learning. The supervisee's assessment also pointed up her healthy interest in knowing what she did not know about intersections in another cultural group. This was explored in later consultations that she sought about race, marriage, power, and stereotyping.

The relationship is illustrative of several important points: it (a) demonstrates the use of consultants recommended by the *Multicultural Guidelines: An Ecological Approach to Context, Identity, and Intersectionality* (APA, 2017b); (b) provides feedback on the developmental nature of supervision (covering early career to established practice); (c) demonstrates the value of cultural humility as an important attitude on the supervisor's part (being able to embrace constructive critical feedback); and (d) addresses the central role that supervision plays in the professional practice cycle.

Other Specialties

Standards to include multicultural competencies are being incorporated and expanded in other specialties and in other countries. For example, the growing recognition of an ever more diverse North America prompted occupational therapists in Canada to accept and understand clients' customs, values, and beliefs so as to realize more effective outcomes. Subsequently, several occupational therapy groups developed a *Joint Position Statement on Diversity* (Association of Canadian Occupational Therapy Regulatory Organizations, the Association of Canadian Occupational Therapy University Programs, the Canadian Association of Occupational Therapists, the Canadian Occupational Therapy Foundation, & the Professional Alliance of Canada, 2007). In it they addressed social justice principles such as the impact of discrimination on access to and engagement in occupations; how sociopolitical factors (e.g., age gender, ability status, religion, citizenship status) influence experiences, values, and opportunities; and whether definitions of well-being that are rooted in White, Western, middle-class cultural values are relevant and valid across all cultures. In their 2014 updated statement (Occupational Therapy Professional Alliance of Canada, 2014), the five organizations strongly encouraged practice, research, education, and theory development in occupational therapy and that they attend to the full range of social and cultural diversity, critically examining biases embedded in the profession, power relations between clients and therapists, power relations within the profession, and connections between individual experiences and broader social structures (p. 1).

Similarly, culturally competent behavior analysts are needed as the number of consumers with diverse backgrounds increases. Fong et al. (2017) explored this need as they addressed the need for relevant academic training to prepare mental health professionals for changing demographics. They identified challenges to training that include "language barriers, negative perceptions about cultures that are different from one's own, microaggressions in work and academic settings, lack of mentoring opportunities, adverse campus climates, and tokenism" (p. 103). Such issues point to the need for more culturally informed curricula and more diverse students and faculty.

MODALITIES

The infusion of multiculturalism with particular methods and procedures of providing psychotherapy is discussed in this section. The modalities described include family therapy, group therapy, couples therapy, and play therapy.

Family Therapy

Taking as a given that all individuals are cultural beings, family, group, and couples therapies must be viewed as cultural systems with all of the complexities that attend to the individual with additional levels of intersectional intricacies. For example, how family is defined varies by cultural identity. Family may comprise cisgender parents and 2.5 children living in a single-family home, or a large multigenerational unit living in a 2-bedroom house on a reservation, or two gender-fluid fathers with adopted children. Does it include ancestors or recently deceased relatives? Zaker and Boostanipoor (2016) stated, "Cultural awareness is a special lens that the family therapist uses to view the client's reality as well as his or her own" (p. 56). Understanding and making good use of a multicultural family's values around the simple concept of "talk" can impact the success of treatment (Zaker & Boostanipoor, 2016). In some cultures, families value talk, while others communicate through other channels such as food. Under what conditions is talk considered inappropriate in terms of relationship status and dynamics? There are myriad multicultural concepts that are interwoven into the tenets of family therapy, including the usual categories. Issues of Western bias in assessments of family expressiveness, autonomy, boundaries, intimacy, and power dynamics are examples. Regarding the latter, Siegel (2016) suggested that certain family therapy approaches fail to focus on oppressive mechanisms such as routine violence (e.g., honor killing) that are sanctioned practices in some cultures and societies.

Group Therapy

Groups, even so-called homogenous groups, are "multicultural," as participants will differ on some aspect of social identity. Miles and Paquin (2014) stated that group leaders must be trained to work ethically and effectively with issues related to diversity and social justice and proposed an essential connection between multicultural and social justice education and evidence-based group practice. D. G. Hays et al. (2010) included community organizing, consciousness-raising, and sociopolitical issues as suitable topics for group work.

Miles et al. (2021) addressed the impact of microaggressions on group dynamics, noting that they should be anticipated given that groups are social microcosms. The group leader has to be vigilant about minimizing harm to the group. This requires the leader to understand systemic inequity and how unchallenged microaggressions perpetuate oppression. Kivlighan et al. (2021) corroborated the frequent occurrence of microaggressions in group therapy and their negative effects on group cohesion. Kivlighan and Chapman (2018) emphasized the importance of the leader intervening in the moment when microaggressions occur to secure a safe and inclusive environment for all. To ensure that oppressed voices are heard, they cautioned against the leader focusing on the person who commits the microaggression, typically individuals who are accustomed to privilege and status and who may respond with fragility, for example, defensiveness.

Kivlighan and Chapman (2018) described how group therapists can use the pillars of multicultural orientation—cultural humility, cultural comfort, and cultural opportunities (described in Chapter 4, this volume)—to establish effective multicultural groups. Arczynski (2017) developed a course that sought to enhance trainees' group therapy multicultural social justice competencies. The course incorporated a number of multicultural assessments, self-evaluations, and seminar discussions among other measures of learning that were determined to be successful in increasing multicultural awareness, knowledge, and skills in their participants.

Couples Therapy

In a chapter in the *APA Handbook of Multicultural Psychology*, Kelly et al. (2014) described cultural competence in couples therapy as a complement to and expansion of multiculturalism. They noted that the best-known empirically supported couples therapy approaches suffered from limitations attendant to a Eurocentric orientation. They posited that cultural competence principles of awareness, knowledge, skills, and dynamic sizing (ability to "flexibly generalize" culture-specific knowledge and to discern when to focus on individual and/or group-based experiences; S. Sue, 2006) attenuate those limitations. Zaker and Boostanipoor (2016), in their recommendations for working with couples, reasoned that a multicultural viewpoint is important as it acknowledges the importance of cultural competencies for couples counselors. Siegel (2016) reported that the number of mixed-race couples has doubled every decade since 1960. Couples therapists have long had to address family of origin issues. The expansion of intermarriage brings with it an increase in the densities of cultural differences that contribute to marital conflict, hence the need for more cultural competence in the therapist (Olver, 2012).

In working with a couple in whom Russian and Lebanese backgrounds came together, Dr. J observed that the levels of intersectionality are intricately multilayered. Intersections of religion, socioeconomic status, education, language, and worldviews must be worked out and negotiated at pivot points impacting parenting, power, and personalities. Kelly et al. (2014), in their handbook entry covering multicultural approaches to couples and marital therapy, discussed culturally competent treatment of diverse couples and pointed out that traditional treatments have notable limitations based on their common Eurocentric orientation.

Play Therapy

There is a seamless fit between multicultural therapy and play therapy. Those who work therapeutically with children understand that play is their work. Interpreting what children bring into the office setting cannot depend solely on language; it may not be well developed, it may be a second language, or it may be withheld. Observing and analyzing the play offers a rich source of information about the child. Knowing something about the child's culture informs the impressions of the play and, hence, understanding of the child. Killian et al. (2017) found in working with Somali refugee children that a multiculturally sensitive approach that considered their culture's collectivist views, the role of Islam, cultural taboos, and more helped them understand and address their specific needs. Shen (2016) surveyed school counselors and found that play therapy facilitated a more positive response from ethnically diverse school children than did talk therapy.

As diversity increases within the country, so too will the need for multiculturally trained therapists, including play therapists, and more research is needed on multicultural play therapy. Yee et al. (2019) analyzed 10 years of publication on play therapy and reported a severe lack of articles with a multicultural focus.

All of these modalities encompass important multicultural considerations. It is incumbent upon leaders and counselors to apply a social justice lens to their work. Diversity within groups, interracial marriage, and cross-cultural families will surface issues of marginalization, privilege, and oppression (Burnes & Ross, 2010).

LICENSING

Components that define effective multicultural therapy have become essential parts of the paradigms of licensing as well. The Examination for Professional Practice in Psychology (EPPP) is designed by the Association of State and Provincial Psychology Boards (ASPPB) for licensing psychologists in the United States and Canada (ASPPB, 2017). Its aim is to assess knowledge that is believed to be critical for the competent practice of psychology. Domain 3 of the exam addresses Social and Cultural Bases of Behavior, constituting 11% of the exam. Models of racial identity (e.g., Black, White, and cross-racial), effects of racial identity in therapy (e.g., therapist/client parallel, progressive, and regressive interactions; and differences in their stages of identity development), and issues of acculturation (e.g., assimilation, integration, marginalization, and separation) are covered (ASPPB, 2017).

The EPPP is designed to assess Part 1—Knowledge, and Part 2—Skills (ASPPB, 2017). Part 2 was added to provide an independent, standardized, reliable, and valid assessment of the demonstrable skills necessary for independent practice.

Domain 3: Relational Competence of the EPPP Part 1 addresses the psychologist's ability "to engage in meaningful and helpful professional relationships, as well as to understand and interact appropriately in a variety of diverse cultural and social contexts. It includes the two sub-categories of diversity and relationships" (ASPPB, 2017, p. 7). The areas related to multicultural competencies assessed by Part 1 are summarized as follows:

- Integrate and apply theory, research, professional guidelines, and personal understanding about social contexts to work effectively with diverse clients
- Work effectively with individuals, families, groups, communities, and/or organizations
- Demonstrate respect for others in all areas of professional practice
- Identify and manage interpersonal conflict between self and others (ASPPB, 2017, pp. 17–18)

These competencies interface well with multicultural therapy concepts and principles that recognize the bidirectional relational influences, acknowledge the importance of empathetic communication, respect differing viewpoints, and value the role of consultation in addressing interpersonal conflict. When certifying entities require demonstration of the ability to "work effectively with diverse clients," to use "culturally appropriate skills, techniques, and behaviors with an appreciation of individual differences," and to work effectively using "relational skills to engage, establish, and maintain working relationships with arrange [sic] of clients" (ASPPB, 2017, p. 17), it reinforces the criticality of infusing multicultural competency skills into the assessment of practice readiness.

The EPPP is not without controversy. Sharpless (2018) reviewed the scores of 4,892 doctoral-level first-time New York EPPP test takers with regard to their gender, ethnicity, and degree type (PhD vs. PsyD). He found that Black examinees had a failure rate of 38.50%, Hispanics had a rate of 35.60%, Asians failed at a 24% rate, and Whites failed at a 14.07% rate. In partial replication study data from another state, Sharpless (2021) reported failure rates of 23.33% for Blacks, 18.60% for Hispanics, 5.75% for Whites, and 3.33% for Asians. Sharpless (2019) recommended more extensive validity testing for both parts of the EPPP given concerns about its criterion and predictive validity. Callahan et al. (2020) contended that the EPPP Part 2's lack of inclusion of certain facets of validity and ASPPB's processes and procedures foster linguistic and racism biases that may have unintended consequences such as restricting diversity in the psychology workforce.

Forum discussions of the controversies elevate other considerations of the data that suggest the need for a deeper dive. Questions arise about the influence of intersecting variables such as abiding systemic racism spanning the preparation spectrum from high school through graduate school, GPA to GRE (Gómez et al., 2021), the quality of training programs, access to practice materials, and APA accreditation. In a private communication with Dr. Matt Turner (June 16, 2021), the senior director of examination services of the ASPPB, Dr. J discussed these questions/concerns. Dr. Turner did not argue the inequities reflected in the Sharpless (2018, 2019, 2021) data, recognizing the national struggle with institutional and systemic racism. ASPPB has identified a pathway to data collection on ethnicity that is in its second year. He shared that ASPPB is a membership organization and cannot compel data collection or sharing. He noted that what is known from historic data is that APA accreditation is a significant variable because they produce examinees with passing rates of 85% compared with a passing rate of 55% for examinees of non-accredited programs.

ASPPB's efforts to ensure against item bias (particularly pertaining to content validity) is facilitated by the Examination Stakeholder Technical Advisory Group, a group of individuals with diverse backgrounds in training, regulatory matters, psychology specialties, measurement, and others, including Dr. Sharpless. Dr. Turner noted that

> a lot of the processes that we [ASPPB] put in place should eliminate or reduce bias; there is a lot of evidence that maybe there is not much bias on this exam. At what point do you do you say maybe this exam is an indicator of not only systemic problems, but something that's going on in training? (M. Turner, personal communication, June 16, 2021)

The EPPP's fidelity to its Domain 3 competencies will inculcate multicultural competencies, the foundation of multicultural therapy, into the assessment of competent practice of psychology.

CONTINUING EDUCATION

The requirement for continuing education (CE) credits by various juris-dictional boards is designed to document efforts to maintain, develop, and increase competencies to improve services to the public and enhance contributions to the profession. Particularly in the field of psychology, ongoing training in ethics is required to protect the rights, welfare, and safety of consumers. Of 62 states, provinces, territories, and the District of Columbia, 34 have such CE requirements with ethics content (CE Classes, 2020). Efforts are being made to ensure that multicultural competence is viewed and valued in the same way, that is, required for the health and protection of the public and enrichment of the profession. The data regarding CE requirements in diversity, cultural competence, or implicit bias for psychologists show that we have a long way to go. As of the publication of this monograph, only seven of 62 states, provinces, territories, and the District of Columbia have such requirements (CE Classes, 2020). Using the state of Oregon as an example, its CE standard endorses a lifelong process of examining values and beliefs and developing and applying an inclusive approach to psychology practice in a manner that recognizes the context and complexities of provider-patient communication and interaction and preserves the dignity of individuals, families, and communities (State of Oregon, Board of Psychology, n.d.).

The effort to require cultural competence continuing education credits for licensure and relicensure has been challenging. As Shashana Koslofsky, a psychologist involved in getting diversity continuing education credits required by legislation in Oregon, reported,

> Here in Oregon, we had a unique approach that was brought on by necessity—our initial attempts to implement this requirement through the Board of Psychology failed. So, we worked with other health professions [and] developed a bill that was passed by the State Legislature. Once the state passed this regulation that Health Professions Boards may require cultural competency CEs, our Board of Psychology was much more willing to implement the requirement. (personal email communication to APA Diversity Listserv, July 22, 2019)

CE requirements for cultural competence and diversity may also impact health disparities. The National Institutes of Health (2017) determined that awareness of, and responsiveness to, differences in patients' cultures are essential in "reducing healthcare disparities and improving access to high-quality healthcare for a diverse group of patients." The U.S. Census Bureau predicts that by 2060 racial and ethnic minorities will increase from 37% to 57% of the population; the total minority population will more than double, from 116.2 million to 241.3 million (U.S. Census Bureau, Public Information Office, 2012). These changes signal the need for greater cognizance of health and treatment disparities and the need for competency in providing care.

The increase in the number of psychologists of color will certainly help advance the evolution and further development of multicultural psychology and multicultural therapy, in particular. As the nation becomes more diverse, so, too, does the pool of mental health professionals. The Center for Workforce Studies at the American Psychological Association (APA, 2018d) reported that from 2007 to 2016 the number of racial and ethnic psychologists almost doubled, increasing by 92%. This represents an increase from 9% to 16% of ethnic minority psychologists in the workforce; the percentage was higher for younger psychologists. Given the historical underrepresentation of racial and ethnic psychologists in the field, it should not be surprising that ethnic minority psychologists tend to be younger (44.7 years) than White psychologists (51.0 years). That the entire spectrum of preparation incorporates multicultural principles should, over time, produce a meaningful number of clinicians who are culturally oriented in multiple spheres. This growth presents an opportunity for racial and ethnic minority psychologists to contribute to the epistemology of psychology as a multicultural discipline.

7

Summary

In review, let us begin with a definition of what multicultural therapy is and is not in the context of psychotherapy theories. A definition of *psychotherapy* that can be applied to most theories was provided by Norcross (1990), as follows:

> Psychotherapy is the informed and intentional application of clinical methods and interpersonal stances derived from established psychological principles for the purpose of assisting people to modify their behaviors, cognitions, emotions, and/or other personal characteristics in directions that the participants deem desirable. (pp. 218–220)

Multicultural therapy, therefore, is the practice of psychotherapy informed by multicultural philosophies and theories grounded in multicultural scholarship on the psychology, race, and ethnicity that leads psychotherapists and their clients toward culturally appropriate strategies

https://doi.org/10.1037/0000279-007
Multicultural Therapy: A Practice Imperative, by M. J. T. Vasquez and J. D. Johnson
Copyright © 2022 by the American Psychological Association. All rights reserved.

and solutions that advance transformation and social change in their lives and in their relationships with their social, emotional, and political environments. It is not an adaptation of other theories/therapies but a complete body of knowledge from which those other systems draw as they evolve to become more appropriate for the Black, Indigenous, People of Color (BIPOC) they serve.

Multicultural competence in psychotherapy has become part of the mainstream fundamental knowledge and skill set required for effective practice. Everyone possesses culturally learned assumptions that influence their life. The multiculturally competent therapist must address the client's culture(s) and be aware of their own in relation to others (American Psychological Association [APA], 2017b; Davis et al., 2018; D. W. Sue & Sue, 2019). Pedersen (2002) proposed that multicultural competence is a three-level developmental sequence: the development of awareness (i.e., appreciation of human cultural diversity leads to cultural sensitivity), knowledge (i.e., factual understanding of basic anthropological knowledge about cultural variation), and skills (i.e., competence and ability to convey cultural empathy). Owen (2013) introduced the concept of "multicultural orientation" (i.e., cultural humility, opportunities and missed opportunities, and cultural comfort) and described it as a "way of being" with the client, while multicultural competencies describe a "way of doing." Cultural humility, "having an interpersonal stance that is other-oriented rather than self-focused, characterized by respect and lack of superiority toward an individual's cultural background and experience" (Hook et al., 2013, p. 1), has wide acceptance as a way of expressing multicultural values. Together, multicultural orientation and competencies describe how well a therapist engages in and implements their multicultural awareness, knowledge, and skills.

As seen in the horrific histories of slavery in America, Native American removal and the reservation system, stealing lands of and murders of Mexicans in the Southwest, Japanese internments, and Hitler's death camps, racism, discrimination, and bias have an enduring and devastating impact that can be felt today. The lasting effects of such oppressive experiences prompted helping and health service professions to include ethical imperatives and practice guidelines that address the importance of competence in psychotherapy, research, and training when working with members of various diverse and/or oppressed groups. The history of mainstream psychology's prejudice and discrimination and the need for affiliation among professionals within cultural, ethnic, and racial groups led to the formation of national ethnic minority psychological associations. Culturally informed psychological science is necessary now more than ever as the nation witnesses more "ingroup" and "outgroup" rhetoric, killing of unarmed BIPOC, defamation of synagogues, and contemporary concentration camps confining Brown and Black refugees and asylum seekers at the southern border.

Because biases reduce one's ability to empathize with others, lawmakers and other policy makers (predominantly White) have historically criminalized people of color. "Law and order" platforms, supposedly race-neutral, use policing as the primary tool for managing mental health and substance use disorders, community problems, and economic inequality. The people in positions to pass and enforce these policies and laws frequently do not see their privilege and reductively attribute other people's "failures" to personal responsibility (i.e., "do the crime, do the time") rather than to the structures and systems that have enabled the maintenance of racial inequities.

Even so-called positive biases, for example, the Asian "model minority," create psychological pressure. As a client of Dr. J confided, "It is difficult to live in a world where even one's parents are ashamed that I went to an ordinary university, obtained ordinary grades, and am still looking for the ideal job." Microaggressions and color-blindness must be monitored for their "death by a thousand cuts" potential.

"Allostatic load" is a helpful construct depicting the combined impact of stressors affecting our minds and bodies (McEwen & Stellar, 1993). As our bodies strive to cope in stressful situations, our neuroendocrine systems discharge high levels of specific hormones. When the stressors are chronic, such as living under the constant fear of deportation or your race being blamed for a viral pandemic, these hormonal fluctuations cause wear and tear on our immune and cardiovascular systems, among others. Acute life events, for example, the illness and death of a loved one, add to one's allostatic load, especially when layered with chronic stressors. The maxim "What doesn't kill you makes you stronger" fails the test in these circumstances, as high allostatic load scores are consistently associated with increased all-cause mortality in adult populations (McEwen & Stellar, 1993). Guidi et al. (2021), in a comprehensive review of the literature, reported high allostatic load associated with ethnicity, perceived racial discrimination, and acculturation stress. They also noted that allostatic overload has been used to conceptualize the physical and psychological states of frontline medical health workers facing the COVID-19 pandemic (Theorell, 2020; Zhang et al., 2020). The stress of confronting the pandemic on a more acute level by those workers makes the cumulative burden of confronting chronic stress coupled with increased risk for contracting the virus for BIPOC, both practitioner and client alike, even more compelling.

The "relationship" has been documented as the key factor in successful therapy, with trust being a key ingredient. Attention is given to the role of the therapist in the relationship. Cultural awareness and knowledge of the client's cultural context are needed to facilitate trust and to accurately convey warmth, genuineness, and empathy in a manner that is meaningful to the client. A multicultural therapist is committed to developing a non-racist identity by first acknowledging that one's racism exists; this requires the tolerance of the unpleasant association with an honest appraisal of one's biases and prejudices (D. W. Sue, 2003).

One of the most important strategies in working with persons of color is to identify their strengths and resilience and use them in the service of their treatment. While we encourage psychotherapists to be aware of barriers, obstacles, and experiences of oppression for clients of color, it is also important to remain open to the strengths and positive aspects of clients' identities. Sometimes adaptations to treatment strategies are necessary, such as incorporating cultural content and values into treatment, using the client's preferred language, and matching clients with therapists of similar ethnicity and race.

In a longer case example, we explored some of the key issues in multi-cultural therapy: dynamics of race and gender differences in dyads, addressing spirituality, initiating discussions about race in the therapy session, dynamics of racial parity in therapeutic dyads, and cultural humility from multiple perspectives. The case demonstrated how a European American therapist's cultural humility allowed her African American male patient to explore his presenting concerns. It enabled her to comfortably refer him to a racially matched therapist and facilitated his return to their work together. Both agreed that her gender, religion, and manner may have prompted the initial contact, but it was her respect for all of his cultural identities that kept him engaged.

Evaluation of multicultural therapy's effectiveness looks at its points of congruence with other forms of therapy, particularly the three acknowledged "forces" of psychodynamic, humanistic, and behavioral therapies. Assessing transference and countertransference issues in the psychodynamic tradition can be viewed as a parallel process to recognizing and understanding that a patient's identity is fluid and multidetermined and that therapist attitudes and beliefs influence clinical and empirical conceptualizations. Humanism's focus on establishing the alliance and viewing behavior in collective and social justice contexts (Comas-Díaz, 2012a) aligns with multicultural awareness and appreciation of individual and cultural differences. Behaviorism's consideration of learned behaviors and how the environment influences those behaviors is akin to the multicultural therapist's consideration of not only immediate environmental variables but also environmental influences in the larger context that includes analysis of available resources.

Even though there are no "natural enemies" of multicultural therapy, there are limitations. Tao et al.'s (2015) meta-analysis using traditional measures of therapeutic processes and outcomes (i.e., working alliance, client satisfaction, general counseling competence, session impact, and symptom improvement) in assessing client ratings of therapist multicultural competencies did not find any significant correlations between multicultural competence and outcome. Researchers such as D. W. Sue and Sue (2016) have pointed out "the plausibility of articulating and measuring MCCs [multicultural competencies]—particularly skills and knowledge—for the entirety of a client's salient and less salient identities becomes untenable" (p. 90).

Intersectionality research, in general, points to the inescapable complexities of addressing all the ways we exist in the world. Ridley, Mollen, et al. (2021) went so far as to declare that multicultural counseling competencies have reached an impasse given the lack of operationalization. After years of dedicated scholarship, there is still a lack of a road map delineating "how" to facilitate therapeutic change. The authors suggested that an integrative model of multicultural competence would include the strengths of the three most prominent models and add the specificity needed to direct the practitioner toward the concrete steps that must be taken on the road to competency.

Many concerns about multicultural therapy are associated with the therapist rather than the therapy. Multicultural therapy must involve a well-trained therapist. Facility with terminology or having had "the" course does not qualify one as a culturally responsive professional. It is a continuous or lifelong endeavor that requires assertive commitment to growth. There are special issues for practitioners of color. We must confront and address the internalized racism that our clients of color bring, as well as the internalized bias that European American clients may bring.

The threads of social justice are inextricably interwoven into the fabric of multicultural therapy. The distinctions between the philosophies, as noted by Ratts and Pedersen (2014), focus on change. Multiculturalism perspectives focus on change within the individual and interpersonal dynamics. Social justice recognizes that living in an unjust system creates many of the problems the individual has to address. Various policies, rules, procedures, and practices in society have resulted in horrible and painful consequences for people of color. Segregated housing, cuts in progressive programs, and biased banking practices are examples of those. Social justice addresses changing the power dynamics, issues of equity, and elimination of oppression in all of its forms. The authors ultimately propose that social justice is a significant and key element of multicultural therapy. Perhaps it can be considered as a Fifth Force, with a salience of its own. Given the imperative to focus on the connection between client problems and larger systemic social barriers, the personal is indeed political.

Social justice demands that we walk the talk of advocacy: attending marches, contacting our legislators and government policy makers, writing editorials, visiting, volunteering, contributing, and voting. It demands that we ensure that our offices and meeting places are barrier free, that we lobby for LGBTQ equality, fight against racist immigration practices, and support religious equity. The multicultural therapist can advocate for social justice, as the saying goes, by "speaking truth to power" and privilege.

Norcross et al. (2002) predicted nearly 2 decades ago that multicultural therapy would be a growing force. Indeed, it has, as it has influenced other therapies, guidelines, and organizational structures. Pedagogical implications highlight opportunities inherent in curricula from the high school through graduate school levels and on to practice that emphasize both individual courses on and infusion of multiculturalism in all courses, training and supervision standards, counseling, research competencies, and more.

The Examination for Professional Practice in Psychology (Association of State and Provincial Psychology Boards, 2017), the licensing examination that is used in most U.S. states and Canadian provinces, assesses a number of culture-based competencies, including models of racial identity, the effects of racial identity in therapy, and issues of acculturation. Building on these assessed competencies and the presumption that continuing education enhances skills, licensing boards can further the cause by requiring cultural competence continuing education credits for licensure and licensure renewals. Lamentably, the number of states, provinces, and territories that have CE requirements in diversity or cultural competence for psychologists is far below what the current zeitgeist demands (http://ce-classes.com/state-requirements-for-psychologists/).

All researchers should become cultural psychologists by seeing the advantages that cultural differences might bring to research. They should seek opportunities for collaboration between the practice and research communities to ensure the most reliable, valid, and generalizable results. The community-based participatory research (CBPR) approach to research with vulnerable populations offers a promising alternative to the traditional "outside-expert" approach. It emphasizes community participation/community voice, community member active and equal participation, methodological rigor, and research team cohesiveness, among other important criteria (Holkup et al., 2004). Paquin et al. (2019) also urged the research psychologist to "actively assume social and personal responsibility for how, what, and why we engage in psychotherapy science" (p. 499).

MULTICULTURAL THERAPY: A SWOT ANALYSIS

Taking a business perspective in evaluating the status and future of multicultural therapy, a strengths, weaknesses, opportunities, and threats (SWOT) analysis may have some utility as we summarize the main theses of this monograph.

Strengths

At a fundamental level, multicultural psychology's major strength is that it lives up to its purpose of providing ethical and effective interventions for culturally diverse clients and advocating for social justice. It has mobilized a generation of practitioners to view their work through a lens of openness and mutual respect and has been a catalyst for change in other areas of theory, practice, training, and research.

There are myriad examples of the infusion of multicultural psychology principles into a variety of systems, programs, organizations, standards, and guidelines. The infusion spans the psychology pedagogical systems from high school through professional practice, and the influence is expanding into other fields of study (Aragón et al., 2017). Preparation for practice in multicultural therapy has benefitted from competency informed guidelines and regulatory mandates. Though it is proceeding at a slow pace, it is important to note that state licensing boards are beginning to require ongoing evidence of training in multicultural therapy principles (e.g., cultural competence). Increasing efforts toward bringing more licensing bodies on board will help ensure that an understanding that cultural contexts of emotion and behavior is essential to effective and ethical interventions for all recipients of mental health services.

Weaknesses

Ridley, Mollen, et al. (2021) exposed some of the fault lines that exist within the multicultural therapy movement. The lack of operational details for becoming culturally competent is a valid complaint. After 50+ years of being a presence and then a force in the psychotherapy world, the movement needs to identify clear prescriptive as well as descriptive mechanisms for operationalizing the competency construct. Consensus on a definition will help anchor the construct and allow for further explication of its principal components. Data will be forthcoming on the success of their model.

Some criticism of multicultural therapy centers on its narrow focus on race and ethnicity, leaving other aspects of identity (e.g., religion, immigration status, ability) not as broadly investigated or addressed; yet we are encouraged by the focus on intersectionality within the multicultural movement. New models might consider factoring in a viewpoint suggested by Goodwin et al. (2018) that multicultural competence may not be a skill that is stable and fixed. They offered instead that it may be fluid, not stably maintained, and varying across patient dyads. Flexibility in responsivity may be appropriate in certain patient contexts. It remains an obligation of all multicultural therapists to ensure that refinement of fundamental constructs is a continuous function of practice informing theory and theory influencing practice.

Opportunities

As the multicultural therapy movement continues to evolve, a question still to be answered is: How should it be inculcated as the "fourth wave" in psychotherapeutic perspectives? Does it imply a "mandate" that all forms of therapy incorporate multicultural concepts into its core principles? Is it even possible to conduct effective therapy of any orientation without consideration of the impact of the unique and intersecting identities of the therapist and patient? More than 25 years ago, Arredondo et al. (1993) suggested that within counseling psychology, providing a cultural context to behavior could potentially elevate multiculturalism from a specialty to a core concept.

Most educational and training guidelines specify multicultural competence as a necessity. How should courses focusing on competencies be structured? Should they be offered as single courses, multiple courses to be taken in conjunction with any training orientation, or a combination of both? Mio (2003) rejected the single course, opting instead for an integrative model, a cluster of courses that cover a wide range of critical cultural concepts, while Michael and Bartoli's (2017) model combined the one course with the infusion approach and multicultural self-awareness labs.

T. B. Smith and Trimble (2016) described multicultural psychology as "a construction project, not a single edifice but a vast complex of buildings. In a word, it is a community, a community in which all are welcomed, none excluded" (p. 246). Clearly, the options are more extensive than viewing it either as a stand-alone theory or infusion into all theories. In any case, there are rich opportunities in developing models that best fit multicultural training competencies. Regardless of the level of offerings, the challenge is to keep the construction going by offering relevant courses, whether this is done by teaching a single course, multiple courses, attending to cultural diversity in all psychology courses, or offering a comprehensive multicultural curriculum. There is an increasingly diverse student population, and it is important to teach appreciation of the central role and relevance of culture. The challenge/opportunity is to keep the movement open to all engineers, lawyers, accountants, teachers, and culinary artists by infusing multiculturalism into all course offerings.

La Roche (2021) suggested that the evolution of several APA guidelines, including the APA *Multicultural Guidelines: An Ecological Approach to Context, Identity, and Intersectionality* (2017b) and the *APA Guidelines on Race and Ethnicity in Psychology: Promoting Responsiveness and Equity* (2019b), helped to advance the conceptualization and practice of culture in psychology, such that they are substantial enough to constitute a paradigmatic shift with significant implications and challenges for the development of evidence-based psychotherapies. He challenged the notion of universal, color-blind interventions *and* treatments designed for racial–ethnic minorities to a more inclusive type of evidence-based psychotherapy that measures and systematically benefits from multiple, changing, and intersecting characteristics (e.g., race, gender orientation, political orientation). He proposed three components of a cultural match model to assist psychologists to conduct more innovative research and clinical work not only with cultural minorities and international communities but with and for all. The continued evolution of multicultural theories and therapy will stimulate evolution of thought, research, and practice.

Threats

A threat can be perceived as anything from the "outside" that can cause harm or vulnerabilities that stem from weaknesses. The "outside," the sociopolitical environment in which one lives, contributes to the level of threat. The unranked list of issues that we all confront includes but is not limited to racial injustice, gun violence, health care, voting rights restrictions, LGBTQ+ rights, body autonomy, refugee crisis and immigration, and climate change, to name a few. Items on the list are fluid; new issues are added or deleted as tensions change. It is important to note that the relevance of items on the list pivots on all of the intersectional factors we have identified. These become critical matters as they are social justice matters. We have noted the inseparable connection between multicultural psychology and social justice. Psychotherapy cannot be relevant or effective if it does not operate in the context of the patient's and psychotherapist's real-world exigencies. Awareness cannot sit dormant; it demands active advocacy. There are forces that actively (White supremacy) or passively (systemic racism, privilege) work against fairness. A lawyer (Beatty, 2020) wrote in an editorial in a Florida newspaper in 2021, "In practice, there is no difference between Marxist government control of all aspects of our lives, and the social justice being advocated today." Racist, homophobic, anti-Semitic, and other hateful rhetoric and actions are a threat to the foundations of multicultural therapy and require imperative action to oppose them.

Threats that arise out of the identified weaknesses are in part ideological. Differences in perspectives on where the movement stands serve to put the movement on notice that there needs to be ongoing assessment of its progress. Is it where it needs to be in terms of developmental stage? What are reasonable expectations of where multicultural psychology should be and along which dimensions? The threat is existential: How will multicultural psychology remain dynamically relevant (proving its effectiveness) in its goals of facilitating therapeutic change while living out its commitment to social justice (demonstrating its commitment)?

The SWOT analysis identifies that multicultural psychology's strength is in its purpose. It is expanding its advocacy efforts by urging licensing boards to include cultural competency in its requirements for ongoing professional proficiency. Abundant opportunities exist to determine the direction the force will take in its emphasis and in developing single, multiple, or broad curriculum courses. Weaknesses center on cultural competence construct diffuseness. New models are being developed that are intended to address a number of perceived deficits. Multicultural therapy would do well to embrace intersectionality and ensure that sufficient attention is given to other areas of identity, because human beings are not unidimensional, and addressing the complexities of our identities may well enhance the therapeutic alliance and treatment outcomes.

CONCLUSION

The force that is multicultural therapy will continue gaining influence. We have documented its impact, revealed its vulnerabilities, and identified its effectiveness. Its synergistic connection with social justice ensures its elevated purpose and imperative action by acknowledging the contexts in which we live and work. We anticipate that new models will evolve that test the fit and precision of competencies that drive multicultural therapy. Research will continue on its applicability and adaptability to more levels of cultural identities and collective experiences of oppression. Given its essentiality to the assurance of effective and respectful treatment of both minority and majority communities, we predict that multicultural therapy will come to be regarded not as exemplary of but as definitive of professional practice.

Glossary of Key Terms

ACCULTURATION   Cultural modification of an individual, group, or people by adapting to or borrowing traits from another culture (e.g., the *acculturation* of immigrants to American life); a merging of cultures as a result of prolonged contact.

ADDRESSING FRAMEWORK   Developed by P. A. Hays (2016), the ADDRESSING model is a framework that facilitates recognition and understanding of the complexities of individual identity. According to Hays, consideration of <u>A</u>ge, developmental <u>D</u>isabilities, acquired <u>D</u>isabilities, <u>R</u>eligion, <u>E</u>thnicity, <u>S</u>exual orientation, <u>S</u>ocioeconomic status, <u>I</u>ndigenous group membership, <u>N</u>ationality, and <u>G</u>ender contributes to a complete understanding of cultural identity.

ALLOSTATIC LOAD   The cumulative adverse effect on the body when subjected to repeated stressors; the cost of chronic exposure to elevated or fluctuating endocrine or neural responses resulting from chronic or repeated challenges that an individual experiences as stressful.

ASSIMILATION   Process through which individuals, groups, and people of differing heritages acquire the habits, attitudes, and modes of life of another culture.

BIPOC   Black, Indigenous, People of Color; while the term *POC* has been widely used as an umbrella term for all people of color, emphasizing Black and Indigenous peoples recognizes that they are disproportionately impacted by systemic and racial injustices.

COGNITIVE SCHEMATA   Concepts and ideas that an individual uses to organize knowledge and guide thought and behavior.

COLLECTIVIST AND INDIVIDUALIST CULTURES   *Collectivist* cultures emphasize family and work group goals above individual needs or desires and value is characterized by emphasis on cohesiveness among individuals and prioritization of the group over the self. *Individualistic* cultures are oriented around the self, being independent instead of identifying with a group mentality. They see each other as only loosely linked and value personal goals over group interests.

COLOR-BLIND IDEOLOGY   The belief that racism is a thing of the past and that race no longer plays a role in understanding people's lived experience. Racial blindness or color-blindness reflects an ideal in the society in which skin color is insignificant. Color-blindness can undermine recognition of the hardships of systemic and institutional oppression of minority groups.

COMMON FACTORS   Those variables considered universal to various types of therapy, such as the therapeutic alliance, that promote therapeutic effectiveness irrespective of theory or intervention employed.

COMMUNITY-PARTNERED PARTICIPATORY RESEARCH (CPPR; also COMMUNITY-BASED PARTICIPATORY RESEARCH [CBPR])   An approach to research that involves collective, reflective, and systematic inquiry in which researchers and community stakeholders engage as equal partners in all steps of the research process with the goals of educating, improving practice, and/or bringing about social change; it questions the power relationships that are inherently embedded in Western knowledge production, advocates for power to be shared between the researcher and the researched, acknowledges the legitimacy of experiential knowledge, and focuses on research aimed at improving lives.

CRITICAL RACE THEORY   A body of scholarship that critically examines how racism and disparate racial outcomes are the result of complex, dynamic, and often subtle social and institutional systems rather than explicit and intentional behavioral practices on the part of individuals.

CULTURAL COMPETENCE   A set of congruent behaviors, attitudes, and policies that come together in a system, agency, or among professionals in their practice that enables effective work in multi- and cross-cultural situations, where *competence* implies having the capacity to function effectively as an individual and an organization within the context of the cultural beliefs, behaviors, and needs presented by consumers and their communities, and includes the following:

CULTURAL EMPATHY   Ability to appreciate experiences of people from other cultures in comparison to one's own.

CULTURAL KNOWLEDGE   Familiarity with the mental parts of a culture, such as beliefs, attitudes, norms, values, symbols, constructions of reality, and worldviews.

CULTURAL SENSITIVITY   Awareness that cultural differences and similarities between people exist without judging or assigning a value, positive or negative, better or worse, right or wrong.

CULTURAL FORMULATION INTERVIEW   Developed by the American Psychiatric Association and the *DSM-5* Cross-Cultural Issues Subgroup, an evidence-based tool composed of a series of questionnaires that assist clinicians in making person-centered cultural assessments to inform diagnosis and treatment planning.

CULTURAL HUMILITY   Process of self-reflection and lifelong inquiry involving awareness of personal and cultural biases as well as cultural competence when interacting with others.

CULTURALLY ADAPTED INTERVENTIONS   Linguistic and cultural modifications of evidence-based treatments or interventions not originally developed to consider language, culture, and context.

EMIC AND ETIC   *Emic* is defined as an insider's account or perspective that is culture specific. The meaning of behavior can only be defined from within the culture studied. *Etic* compares cultural phenomena across cultures. It assumes underlying psychological mechanisms are universal across cultures.

EMOTIONAL EMANCIPATION CIRCLES   Evidence-informed, culturally grounded self-help support groups in which Black people share stories and deepen their understanding of the impact of historical forces and their sense of self-worth. Originated by the Community Healing Network and developed in collaboration with the Association of Black Psychologists (ABPsi), they are designed to help heal, and end, the trauma caused by anti-Black racism.

EMPIRICALLY SUPPORTED TREATMENT (also EVIDENCE-BASED PRACTICE)   Treatments and therapies that have research-based medical and scientific evidence showing that they work for the populations studied under the conditions studied.

ETHNICITY   A grouping of people who identify with each other based on shared attributes that distinguish them from other groups such as a common set of traditions, ancestry, language, history, society, culture, nation, religion, or social treatment within their residing area.

ETHNOCENTRICITY   A belief in the inherent superiority of one's own ethnic group or culture.

FAMILISMO   A concept and value within Latinx cultures that describe the family structure and the importance of family relationships.

GUIDELINES   Aspirational in intent, pronouncements, statements, or declarations that suggest or recommend specific professional behavior, endeavor, or conduct.

CLINICAL GUIDELINES   Recommendations based on independent systematic reviews of the research on treatments for specific disorders or health conditions.

PROFESSIONAL GUIDELINES   Supported by scholarly literature, designed to guide practitioners regarding roles, populations, or settings.

HISPANIC (also LATINX) PARADOX   An epidemiological phenomenon referring to the findings that Hispanic and Latinx peoples tend to have health outcomes that "paradoxically" are comparable to, or in some cases better than, those of their U.S. non-Hispanic White counterparts, even though Hispanic and Latinx people living in the United States have lower average income and education.

IMPLICIT BIAS   A bias or prejudice that is present but not consciously held or recognized.

INTERSECTIONALITY (also INTERSECTIONAL IDENTITIES)   A framework for understanding how social identities (e.g., gender, race, ethnicity, social class, religion, sexual orientation, ability, and gender identity) overlap with one another and with systems of power that oppress and advantage people in different contexts.

MICROAGGRESSION   A statement, action, or incident regarded as an instance of indirect, subtle, or unintentional discrimination against members of marginalized groups.

MODEL MINORITY   A minority demographic whose members are stereotypically perceived to achieve a higher degree of socioeconomic success than the population average.

MULTICULTURAL COMPETENCE   Obtaining the awareness, knowledge, and skills to work with people of diverse backgrounds in an effective manner.

MULTICULTURAL ORIENTATION   Examines how cultural worldviews, values, and beliefs of the client and therapist interact and influence one another to cocreate a relational experience in the spirit of healing.

MULTICULTURAL PSYCHOLOGY   An extension of general psychology that recognizes that multiple aspects of identity influence a person's worldview, including race, ethnicity, language, sexual orientation, gender, age, disability, class status, education, religious or spiritual orientation, and other cultural dimensions, and that both universal and culture-specific phenomena should be taken into consideration when psychologists are helping clients, training students, advocating for social change and justice, and conducting research.

MULTICULTURAL RESPONSIVENESS   The ability to learn from and relate respectfully with people of one's own culture as well as those from other cultures.

MULTICULTURAL THERAPY   Any form of psychotherapy that considers the clients' multiple aspects of identity; the potential cultural bias (e.g., racism, sexism) of the practitioner; the history of oppressed and marginalized groups; acculturation issues for immigrant clients; and the politics of power as they affect clients.

RACE   Grouping of humans based on shared physical or social qualities into categories generally viewed as distinct by society.

RACIAL DISPARITIES   The imbalances and incongruities between treatments or outcomes for racial groups, including economic status, income, housing options, medical treatment, societal treatment, safety and violence, and myriad other aspects of life and society.

RACISM   Prejudice, discrimination, or antagonism directed against a person or people based on racial or ethnic group membership, typically one that is a minority or marginalized.

AVERSIVE RACISM   A form of racial prejudice felt by individuals who outwardly endorse egalitarian attitudes and values but nonetheless experience negative emotions or exhibit discriminatory practices, in the presence of members of certain racial groups, particularly in ambiguous circumstances.

INTERNALIZED RACISM   The personal conscious or subconscious acceptance of the dominant society's racist views, stereotypes, and biases of one's racial and/or ethnic group.

STRUCTURAL RACISM (also INSTITUTIONAL AND SYSTEMIC)   A system in which public policies, institutional practices, and other norms work in ways to reinforce and perpetuate racial inequities.

SOCIAL JUSTICE   The view that everyone deserves equal economic, political, legal, and social rights, experiences, and opportunities.

SOCIAL LOCATION   The many intersections of our experience related to race, religion, age, physical size, sexual orientation, social class, and so on within any given context.

STEREOTYPE THREAT   A perceived psychological threat arising from when one is in a situation for which a negative stereotype about one's group applies.

SWOT ANALYSIS   A study undertaken by an organization to identify its internal Strengths and Weaknesses as well as its external Opportunities and Threats.

THERAPEUTIC ALLIANCE (also WORKING ALLIANCE)   The cooperative working relationship between the client and therapist featuring mutual respect and shared goals; considered as essential to effective treatment.

UNCONSCIOUS BIAS (also UNCONSCIOUS RACIAL STEREO-
   TYPES)   Stereotypes about certain groups of people that individuals
   form outside their own conscious awareness.

WEIRD PARTICIPANT SAMPLES   Research samples drawn from
   populations that are White, Educated, Industrialized, Rich, and
   Democratic. Ninety-nine percent of all published studies rely on
   participants recruited from populations that share these qualities.

WORKING MEMORY   The small amount of information that can be
   held in an especially accessible state and used in cognitive tasks.

   CULTURAL WORKING MEMORY   Coined by Dr. Josephine
   Johnson in this monograph, the acquisition of factual knowledge
   of relevant cultural factors before applying it in individual, meaningful, and fluid ways within the psychotherapeutic relationship.

Suggested Readings

In addition to the works we cite in this monograph, your journeys toward becoming multiculturally competent clinicians may also be informed by the following works:

American Psychological Association, Society for the Teaching of Psychology (n.d.). *Presidential Taskforce on Diversity Education* [Resources]. http://teachpsych.org/diversity/ptde/index.php

Bryant-Davis, T. (2019). *Multicultural feminist therapy: Helping adolescent girls of color to thrive*. American Psychological Association.

Helms, J. E. (2020). *A race is a nice thing to have: A guide to being a White person or understanding the White persons in your life* (3rd ed.). Cognella Academic Publishing.

Ibrahim, F. A., & Heuer, J. T. (2016). *Cultural and social justice counseling: Client-specific interventions*. Springer International Publishing.

Kendi, I. X. (2019). *How to be an antiracist*. Random House.

Korn, L. E. (2016). *Multicultural counseling workbook: Exercises, worksheets & games to build rapport with diverse clients*. PESI Publishing & Media.

McGhee, H. (2021). *The sum of us: What racism costs everyone and how we can prosper together*. One World.

Obama, B. (2020). *A promised land*. Random House.

Obama, M. (2018). *Becoming*. Random House.

Pedersen, P. B., Lonner, W. J., Draguns, J. G., Trimble, J. E., & Scharron-del Rio, M. R. (Eds). (2016). *Counseling across cultures* (7th ed.). Sage.

Soto, A., Smith, T. B., Griner, D., Domenech-Rodríguez, M., & Bernal, G. (2018). Cultural adaptations and therapist multicultural competence: Two meta-analytic reviews. *Journal of Clinical Psychology, 74*(11), 1907–1923. https://doi.org/10.1002/jclp.22679

Sue, D. W. (2016). *Race talk and the conspiracy of silence: Understanding and facilitating difficult dialogues on race.* John Wiley & Sons.

Wilkerson, I. (2020). *Caste: The origins of our discontents.* Random House.

References

Abramson, A. (2021). How to overcome imposter syndrome. *Monitor on Psychology*, *52*(4). https://www.apa.org/monitor/2021/06/cover-impostor-phenomenon

Ackerman, S. J., & Hilsenroth, M. J. (2003). A review of therapist characteristics and techniques positively impacting the therapeutic alliance. *Clinical Psychology Review*, *23*(1), 1–33. https://doi.org/10.1016/S0272-7358(02)00146-0

Agency for Healthcare Research and Quality. (2018). *National healthcare quality and disparities reports*. https://www.ahrq.gov/research/findings/nhqrdr/index.html

Aisenberg, E. (2008). Evidence-based practice in mental health care to ethnic minority communities: Has its practice fallen short of its evidence? *Social Work*, *53*(4), 297–306. https://doi.org/10.1093/sw/53.4.297

Allport, G. W. (1954). *The nature of prejudice*. Addison-Wesley.

American Counseling Association. (2003). *American Counseling Association advocacy competencies* (updated 2018). https://www.counseling.org/docs/default-source/competencies/aca-advocacy-competencies-updated-may-2020.pdf?sfvrsn=f410212c_4

American Counseling Association. (2014). *2014 ACA code of ethics*. https://www.counseling.org/docs/default-source/default-document-library/2014-code-of-ethics-finaladdress.pdf

American Counseling Association. (2015). *Multicultural and social justice counseling competencies*. https://www.counseling.org/docs/default-source/competencies/multicultural-and-social-justice-counseling-competencies.pdf?sfvrsn=8573422c_22

American Humanistic Association. (n.d.). *Definition of humanism*. https://americanhumanist.org/what-is-humanism/definition-of-humanism/

American Psychiatric Association. (2013). Cultural formulation. In *Diagnostic and statistical manual of mental disorders* (5th ed., pp. 749–759).

American Psychiatric Association. (2021, January). *APA's apology to Black, Indigenous and People of Color for its support of structural racism in psychiatry.* https://www.psychiatry.org/newsroom/apa-apology-for-its-support-of-structural-racism-in-psychiatry

American Psychological Association. (n.d.). *APA amicus briefs by issue.* https://www.apa.org/about/offices/ogc/amicus/index-issues

American Psychological Association. (2003). Guidelines on multicultural education, training, research, practice, and organizational change for psychologists. *American Psychologist, 58*(5), 377–402. https://doi.org/10.1037/0003-066X.58.5.377

American Psychological Association. (2011a). *Guidelines for assessment of and intervention with persons with disabilities.* http://www.apa.org/pi/disability/resources/assessment-disabilities.aspx

American Psychological Association. (2011b). *National standards for high school psychology curricula.* https://www.apa.org/education-career/k12/psychology-curricula.pdf

American Psychological Association. (2012). Guidelines for psychological practice with lesbian, gay, and bisexual clients. *American Psychologist, 67*(1), 10–42. https://doi.org/10.1037/a0024659

American Psychological Association. (2013). *APA guidelines for the undergraduate psychology major: Version 2.0.* https://www.apa.org/ed/precollege/about/psymajor-guidelines.pdf

American Psychological Association. (2014a). *APA guidelines for clinical supervision in health service psychology.* https://www.apa.org/about/policy/guidelines-supervision.pdf

American Psychological Association. (2014b). Guidelines for psychological practice with older adults. *American Psychologist, 69*(1), 34–65. https://doi.org/10.1037/a0035063

American Psychological Association. (2015a). Guidelines for psychological practice with transgender and gender nonconforming people. *American Psychologist, 70*(9), 832–864. https://doi.org/10.1037/a0039906

American Psychological Association. (2015b). *Standards of accreditation for health service psychology.* https://irp-cdn.multiscreensite.com/a14f9462/files/uploaded/APA-Principles-Accreditation-SoA-AOP_200116.pdf

American Psychological Association. (2016). *2015 APA survey of psychology health service providers.* https://www.apa.org/workforce/publications/15-health-service-providers/

American Psychological Association. (2017a). *Ethical principles of psychologists and code of conduct* (2002, amended effective June 1, 2010, and January 1, 2017). https://www.apa.org/ethics/code/

American Psychological Association. (2017b). *Multicultural guidelines: An ecological approach to context, identity, and intersectionality.* https://www.apa.org/about/policy/multicultural-guidelines.pdf

American Psychological Association. (2018a). *APA guidelines for psychological practice with boys and men.* https://www.apa.org/about/policy/boys-men-practice-guidelines.pdf

American Psychological Association. (2018b). *APA guidelines for psychological practice with girls and women.* https://www.apa.org/about/policy/psychological-practice-girls-women.pdf

American Psychological Association. (2018c). *APA guidelines on core learning goals for master's degree graduates in psychology.* http://www.apa.org/about/policy/masters-goals-guidelines.pdf

American Psychological Association. (2018d). *Demographics of the U.S. psychology workforce: Findings from the 2007–16 American Community Survey.* https://www.apa.org/workforce/publications/16-demographics/report.pdf

American Psychological Association. (2019a). *APA guidelines for psychological practice for people with low-income and economic marginalization.* https://www.apa.org/about/policy/guidelines-low-income.pdf

American Psychological Association. (2019b). *APA guidelines on race and ethnicity in psychology: Promoting responsiveness and equity.* https://www.apa.org/about/policy/guidelines-race-ethnicity.pdf

American Psychological Association, Presidential Task Force on Evidence-Based Practice. (2006). Evidence-based practice in psychology. *American Psychologist, 61*(4), 271–285. https://doi.org/10.1037/0003-066X.61.4.271

Anderson, K. N., Bautista, C. L., & Hope, D. A. (2019). Therapeutic alliance, cultural competence and minority status in premature termination of psychotherapy. *American Journal of Orthopsychiatry, 89*(1), 104–114. https://doi.org/10.1037/ort0000342

Andrasfay, T., & Goldman, N. (2021). Reductions in 2020 US life expectancy due to COVID-19 and the disproportionate impact on the Black and Latino populations. *Proceedings of the National Academy of Sciences, 118*(5), e2014746118. https://doi.org/10.1073/pnas.2014746118

Ani, M. (1994). *Yurugu: An African centered critique of European cultural thought and behavior.* African World Press.

Anyon, Y., Lechuga, C., Ortega, D., Downing, B., Greer, E., & Simmons, J. (2018). An exploration of the relationships between student racial background and the school sub-contexts of office discipline referrals: A critical race theory analysis. *Race, Ethnicity and Education, 21*(3), 390–406. https://doi.org/10.1080/13613324.2017.1328594

Apfelbaum, E. P., Sommers, S. R., & Norton, M. I. (2008). Seeing race and seeming racist? Evaluating strategic colorblindness in social interaction. *Journal of Personality and Social Psychology, 95*(4), 918–932. https://doi.org/10.1037/a0011990

Aragón, O., Dovidio, J., & Graham, M. (2017). Colorblind and multicultural ideologies are associated with faculty adoption of inclusive teaching practices. *Journal of Diversity in Higher Education, 10*(3), 201–215. https://doi.org/10.1037/dhe0000026

Arczynski, A. V. (2017). Multicultural social justice group psychotherapy training: Curriculum development and pilot. *Training and Education in Professional Psychology, 11*(4), 227–234. https://doi.org/10.1037/tep0000161

Arias, E. (2016). *Changes in life expectancy by race and Hispanic origin in the United States, 2013–2014* (NCHS Data Brief No. 244). National Center for Health Statistics. https://www.cdc.gov/nchs/products/databriefs/db244.htm

Arredondo, P., Psalti, A., & Cella, K. (1993). The woman factor in multicultural counseling. *Counseling and Human Development, 25,* 1–8.

Asakura, K., & Maurer, K. (2018). Attending to social justice in clinical social work: Supervision as a pedagogical space. *Clinical Social Work Journal, 46*(4), 289–297. https://doi.org/10.1007/s10615-018-0667-4

Asian American Psychological Association. (2020). *COVID 19 statement.* https://aapaonline.org/wp-content/uploads/2020/04/AAPA-COVID19-statement.pdf

Asnaani, A., & Hofmann, S. G. (2012). Collaboration in multicultural therapy: Establishing a strong therapeutic alliance across cultural lines. *Journal of Clinical Psychology, 68*(2), 187–197. https://doi.org/10.1002/jclp.21829

Association of Canadian Occupational Therapy Regulatory Organizations, the Association of Canadian Occupational Therapy University Programs, the Canadian Association of Occupational Therapists, the Canadian Occupational Therapy Foundation, & the Professional Alliance of Canada. (2007). *Joint position statement on diversity.* https://cotbc.org/wp-content/uploads/JointPS_Diversity.pdf

Association of State and Provincial Psychology Boards. (2017). *The EPPP (Part 2-Skills): The assessment of skills needed for the independent practice of psychology.* https://cdn.ymaws.com/www.asppb.net/resource/resmgr/eppp_2/updated_overview.pdf

Atkin, A. L., Yoo, H., Jager, J., & Yeh, C. J. (2018). Internalization of the model minority myth, school racial composition, and psychological distress among Asian American adolescents. *Asian American Journal of Psychology, 9*(2), 108–116. https://doi.org/10.1037/aap0000096

Atkinson, R. C., & Shiffrin, R. M. (1968). Human memory: A proposed system and its control processes. In K. W. Spence (Ed.), *The psychology of learning and motivation: Advances in research and theory* (pp. 89–195). Academic Press. https://doi.org/10.1016/S0079-7421(08)60422-3

Baddeley, A. (2000). The episodic buffer: A new component of working memory? *Trends in Cognitive Sciences, 4*(11), 417–423. https://doi.org/10.1016/S1364-6613(00)01538-2

Bajaj, S. S., & Stanford, F. C. (2021). Beyond Tuskegee—Vaccine distrust and everyday racism. *The New England Journal of Medicine, 384*(5), e12. https://doi.org/10.1056/NEJMpv2035827

Bareilles, S., & McKenna, L. (2019). A safe place to land. *Amidst the chaos*. Epic Records.

Barile, J., Edwards, V., Dhingra, S., & Thompson, W. (2014). Associations among county-level social determinants of health, child maltreatment, and emotional support on health-related quality of life in adulthood. *Psychology of Violence, 5*(2), 183–191. https://doi.org/10.1037/a0038202

Barnett, J. E., & Johnson, W. B. (2011). Integrating spirituality and religion into psychotherapy: Persistent dilemmas, ethical issues, and a proposed decision-making process. *Ethics & Behavior, 21*(2), 147–164. https://doi.org/10.1080/10508422.2011.551471

Barnett, J. E., Lazarus, A. A., Vasquez, M. J. T., Moorehead-Slaughter, O., & Johnson, W. B. (2007). Boundary issues and multiple relationships: Fantasy and reality. *Professional Psychology: Research and Practice, 38*(4), 401–410. https://doi.org/10.1037/0735-7028.38.4.401

Batson, C. D., Chang, J., Orr, R., & Rowland, J. (2002). Empathy, attitudes, and action: Can feeling for a member of a stigmatized group motivate one to help the group? *Personality and Social Psychology Bulletin, 28*(12), 1656–1666. https://doi.org/10.1177/014616702237647

Beatty, G. (2020, March 20). Push for "social justice" is a threat to free society [Opinion]. *Florida Today*. https://www.floridatoday.com/story/opinion/2020/03/20/push-social-justice-threat-free-society/2886782001/

Behnke, S. (2013, September). *When diversities clash: Sexual orientation, religious beliefs, professional ethics, and the U.S. Constitution* [Conference session]. American Psychological Association Education Leadership Conference, Washington, DC, United States. https://doi.org/10.1037/e633852013-001

Bennett, D., Lee, J., & Cahlan, S. (2020, May 30). The death of George Floyd: What video and other records show about his final minutes. *The Washington Post*. https://www.washingtonpost.com/nation/2020/05/30/video-timeline-george-floyd-death/

Berger, L. K., Zane, N., & Hwang, W.-C. (2014). Therapist ethnicity and treatment orientation differences in multicultural counseling competencies. *Asian American Journal of Psychology, 5*(1), 53–65. https://doi.org/10.1037/a0036178

Bernal, G., & Domenech Rodriguez, M. M. (Eds.). (2012). *Cultural adaptations: Tools for evidence-based practice with diverse populations.* American Psychological Association. https://doi.org/10.1037/13752-000

Bernal, G., Trimble, J. E., Burlew, A. K., & Leong, F. T. L. (Eds.). (2003). *Handbook of racial and ethnic minority psychology.* Sage.

Bernard, J. M., & Goodyear, R. K. (2014). *Fundamentals of clinical supervision* (5th ed.). Merrill.

Bhatia, S. (2002). Acculturation, dialogical voices and the construction of the diasporic self. *Theory & Psychology, 12*(1), 55–77. https://doi.org/10.1177/0959354302121004

Biever, J. L., Castaño, M. T., de las Fuentes, C., González, C., Servín-López, S., Sprowls, C., & Tripp, C. G. (2002). The role of language in training psychologists to work with Hispanic clients. *Professional Psychology: Research and Practice, 33*(3), 330–336. https://doi.org/10.1037/0735-7028.33.3.330

Biever, J. L., Gómez, J. P., González, C. G., & Patrizio, N. (2011). Psychological services to Spanish-speaking populations: A model curriculum for training competent professionals. *Training and Education in Professional Psychology, 5*(2), 81–87. https://doi.org/10.1037/a0023535

The BIPOC Project. (2020, August). *A Black, Indigenous & People of Color movement: About us.* https://www.thebipocproject.org/what-we-do

Blair, C., & Raver, C. C. (2016). Poverty, stress, and brain development: New directions for prevention and intervention. *Academic Pediatrics, 16*(3 Suppl.), S30–S36. https://doi.org/10.1016/j.acap.2016.01.010

Bogart, L. M., Dale, S. K., Daffin, G. K., Patel, K. N., Klein, D. J., Mayer, K. H., & Pantalone, D. W. (2018). Pilot intervention for discrimination-related coping among HIV-positive Black sexual minority men. *Cultural Diversity & Ethnic Minority Psychology, 24*(4), 541–551. https://doi.org/10.1037/cdp0000205

Bohart, A. C., Elliot, R., Greenberg, L. S., & Watson, J. C. (2002). Empathy. In J. C. Norcross (Ed.), *Psychotherapy relationships that work: Therapist contributions and responsiveness to patients* (pp. 89–108). Oxford University Press.

Brief of Amicus Curiae American Psychological Association, American Psychiatric Association, American Association for Marriage and Family Therapy, Georgia Psychological Association, Michigan Psychological Association, & New York State Psychological Association as amici curiae in support of the employees, Bostock v. Clayton County, 590 U.S. ___ (2020) (No. 17-1618). https://www.supremecourt.gov/DocketPDF/17/17-1618/107154/20190703162955652_17-1618%2017-1623%2018-107%20tsac%20APA.pdf

Broadbent, D. E. (1958). *Perception and communication.* Pergamon Press. https://doi.org/10.1037/10037-000

Brown, D. L. (2008). African American resilience: Examining racial socialization and social support as protective factors. *The Journal of Black Psychology, 34*(1), 32–48. https://doi.org/10.1177/0095798407310538

Brown, L. S. (1994). *Subversive dialogues: Theory in feminist therapy.* Basic Books.

Brown, L. S. (2009). Cultural competence: A new way of thinking about integration in therapy. *Journal of Psychotherapy Integration, 19*(4), 340–353. https://doi.org/10.1037/a0017967

Brown, L. S. (2016). *Supervision essentials for the feminist psychotherapy model of supervision.* American Psychological Association. https://doi.org/10.1037/14878-000

Brown v. Board of Education, 347 U.S. 483 (1954). https://www.oyez.org/cases/1940-1955/347us483

Bruneau, E. G., & Saxe, R. (2012). The power of being heard: The benefits of "perspective-giving" in the context of intergroup conflict. *Journal of Experimental Social Psychology, 48*(4), 855–866. https://doi.org/10.1016/j.jesp.2012.02.017

Burnes, T., & Ross, K. (2010). Applying social justice to oppression and marginalization in group process: Interventions and strategies for group counselors. *Journal for Specialists in Group Work, 35*(2), 169–176. https://doi.org/10.1080/01933921003706014

Butler, S. M., & Sheriff, N. (2020, November). *Innovative solutions to address the mental health crisis: Shifting away from police as first responders.* https://www.brookings.edu/research/innovative-solutions-to-address-the-mental-health-crisis-shifting-away-from-police-as-first-responders/

Cabral, R. R., & Smith, T. B. (2011). Racial/ethnic matching of clients and therapists in mental health services: A meta-analytic review of preferences, perceptions, and outcomes. *Journal of Counseling Psychology, 58*(4), 537–554. https://doi.org/10.1037/a0025266

California State University. (2020, July 22). *CSU trustees approve ethnic studies and social justice general education requirement.* https://www2.calstate.edu/csu-system/news/Pages/CSU-Trustees-Approve-Ethnic-Studies-and-Social-Justice-General-Education-Requirement.aspx

Callahan, J. L., Bell, D. J., Davila, J., Johnson, S. L., Strauman, T. J., & Yee, C. M. (2020). The enhanced examination for professional practice in psychology: A viable approach? *American Psychologist, 75*(1), 52–65. https://doi.org/10.1037/amp0000586

Canadian Mental Health Association. (2018, September). *Mental health in the balance: Ending the health care disparity in Canada.* https://cmha.ca/wp-content/uploads/2021/07/CMHA-Parity-Paper-Full-Report-EN.pdf

Captari, L. E., Hook, J. N., Hoyt, W., Davis, D. E., McElroy-Heltzel, S. E., & Worthington, E. L., Jr. (2018). Integrating clients' religion and spirituality within psychotherapy: A comprehensive meta-analysis. *Journal of Clinical Psychology, 74*(11), 1938–1951. https://doi.org/10.1002/jclp.22681

Carlson, J., & Englar-Carlson, M. (2010). Series preface. In L. S. Brown (Ed.), *Feminist therapy* (pp. ix–xii). American Psychological Association.

Casas, J. M., Vasquez, M. J. T., & Ruiz de Esparza, C. A. (2002). Counseling the Latina/o: A guiding framework for a diverse population. In P. B. Pedersen, J. G. Draguns, W. J. Lonner, & J. E. Trimble (Eds.), *Counseling across cultures* (5th ed., pp. 133–160). Sage.

Ceballos, P., Parikh, S., & Post, P. (2012). Examining social justice attitudes among play therapists: Implications for multicultural supervision and training. *International Journal of Play Therapy, 21*(4), 232–243. https://doi.org/10.1037/a0028540

CE Classes. (2020). *State requirements for psychologists.* http://ce-classes.com/state-requirements-for-psychologists/

Centers for Disease Control and Prevention. (2020a, December 10). *Disparities in COVID-19 illness: Racial and ethnic health disparities.* https://www.cdc.gov/coronavirus/2019-ncov/community/health-equity/racial-ethnic-disparities/increased-risk-illness.html

Centers for Disease Control and Prevention. (2020b, December 10). *Disparities in deaths from COVID-19: Racial and ethnic health disparities.* https://www.cdc.gov/coronavirus/2019-ncov/community/health-equity/racial-ethnic-disparities/disparities-deaths.html

Centers for Disease Control and Prevention. (2020c, December 10). *Risk of exposure to COVID-19: Racial and ethnic health disparities.* https://www.cdc.gov/coronavirus/2019-ncov/community/health-equity/racial-ethnic-disparities/increased-risk-exposure.html#:~:text=Neighborhood%20and%20physical%20environment%3A,may%20vary%20between%20counties

Centers for Disease Control and Prevention. (2021, April 22). *Tuskegee Study—Timeline—CDC—NCHHSTP.* Centers for Disease Control and Prevention. https://www.cdc.gov/tuskegee/timeline.htm

Chaudhry, I., Neelam, K., Duddu, V., & Husain, N. (2008). Ethnicity and psychopharmacology. *Journal of Psychopharmacology, 22*(6), 673–680. https://doi.org/10.1177/0269881107082105

Cherry, K. (2020). *Sigmund Freud's theories about religion.* Verywell Mind. https://www.verywellmind.com/freud-religion-2795858

Chiao, J. Y., Cheon, B. K., Pornpattanangkul, N., Mrazek, A. J., & Blizinsky, K. D. (2013). Cultural neuroscience: Progress and promise. *Psychological Inquiry, 24*(1), 1–19. https://doi.org/10.1080/1047840X.2013.752715

Chin, J. L. (2020, March 17). Crisis leadership: The coronavirus pandemic and xenophobia [Blog post]. *Psychology Today.* https://www.psychologytoday.com/us/blog/leadership/202003/crisis-leadership-the-coronavirus-pandemic-and-xenophobia?amp&__twitter_impression=true

Choi, S. A., & Hastings, J. F. (2019). Religion, spirituality, coping, and resilience among African Americans with diabetes. *Journal of Religion & Spirituality in Social Work, 38*(1), 93–114. https://doi.org/10.1080/15426432.2018.1524735

Civil Rights Act of 1964 § 7, 42 U.S.C. § 2000e et seq (1964).

Clark, K. B., & Clark, M. P. (1939). The development of consciousness of self and the emergence of racial identification in Negro preschool children. *The Journal of Social Psychology, 10*(4), 591–599. https://doi.org/10.1080/00224545.1939.9713394

Clarke, C. (2020, July 2). *BIPOC: What does it mean and where did it come from?* CBS News. https://www.cbsnews.com/news/bipoc-meaning-where-does-it-come-from-2020-04-02/

CNN. (2016, July 25). *Michele Obama: "When they go low, we go high"* [Video]. https://www.youtube.com/watch?v=mu_hCThhzWU

Coates, T. (2015). *Between the world and me.* Spiegel & Brau.

Cohen, A. (2016). *Imbeciles: The Supreme Court, American eugenics, and the sterilization of Carrie Buck.* Penguin Press.

Cokley, K. (2021, July 6). Teaching critical race theory is patriotic, not anti-American. *USA Today.* https://static1.squarespace.com/static/55ddf084e4b0f50508acfc5b/t/60e74b57df2ab36408c99425/1625770839895/Teaching+Critical+Race+Theory+is+Patriotic%2C+Not+Anti-American.pdf

Cokley, K., Smith, L., Bernard, D., Hurst, A., Jackson, S., Stone, S., Awosogba, O., Saucer, C., Bailey, M., & Roberts, D. (2017). Impostor feelings as a moderator and mediator of the relationship between perceived discrimination and mental health among racial/ethnic minority college students. *Journal of Counseling Psychology, 64*(2), 141–154. https://doi.org/10.1037/cou0000198

Cole, E. R. (2009). Intersectionality and research in psychology. *American Psychologist, 64*(3), 170–180. https://doi.org/10.1037/a0014564

Comas-Díaz, L. (2006). Cultural variation in the therapeutic relationship. In C. D. Goodheart, A. E. Kazdin, & R. J. Sternberg (Eds.), *Evidence-based psychotherapy: Where practice and research meet* (pp. 81–105). American Psychological Association. https://doi.org/10.1037/11423-004

Comas-Díaz, L. (2012a). Humanism and multiculturalism: An evolutionary alliance. *Psychotherapy: Theory, Research, & Practice, 49*(4), 437–441. https://doi.org/10.1037/a0027126

Comas-Díaz, L. (2012b). Psychotherapy as a healing practice, scientific endeavor, and social justice action. *Psychotherapy: Theory, Research, & Practice, 49*(4), 473–474. https://doi.org/10.1037/a0027820

Comas-Díaz, L., & Jacobsen, F. M. (1991). Ethnocultural transference and countertransference in the therapeutic dyad. *American Journal of Orthopsychiatry, 61*(3), 392–402. https://doi.org/10.1037/h0079267

Comas-Díaz, L., & Jacobsen, F. M. (1995). The therapist of color and the White patient dyad: Contradictions and recognitions. *Cultural Diversity and Mental Health, 1*(2), 93–106. https://doi.org/10.1037/1099-9809.1.2.93

Comas-Díaz, L., & Torres Rivera, E. (Eds.). (2020). *Liberation psychology: Theory, method, practice and social justice.* American Psychological Association. https://doi.org/10.1037/0000198-000

Community Healing Network. (n.d.). *Emotional emancipation circles.* https://communityhealingnet.org/emotional-emancipation-circle/

Connolly Gibbons, M. B., Rothbard, A., Farris, K. D., Stirman, S. W., Thompson, S. M., Scott, K., Heintz, L. E., Gallop, R., & Crits-Christoph, P. (2011). Changes in psychotherapy utilization among consumers of services for major depressive disorder in the community mental health system. *Administration and Policy in Mental Health, 38*(6), 495–503. https://doi.org/10.1007/s10488-011-0336-1

Constantine, M. G. (1998). Developing competence in multicultural assessment: Implications for counseling psychology training and practice. *The Counseling Psychologist, 26*(6), 922–929. https://doi.org/10.1177/0011000098266003

Constantine, M. G. (2001). Predictors of observer ratings of multicultural competence in Black, Latino, and White American trainees. *Journal of Counseling Psychology, 48*(4), 456–462. https://doi.org/10.1037/0022-0167.48.4.456

Cordes, J., & Castro, M. C. (2020). Spatial analysis of COVID-19 clusters and contextual factors in New York City. *Spatial and Spatio-temporal Epidemiology, 34,* 100355. https://doi.org/10.1016/j.sste.2020.100355

Corey, G., & Herlihy, B. (2015). *Boundary issues in counseling: Multiple roles and responsibilities.* American Counseling Association.

Corrigan, P. W., & Salzer, M. S. (2003). The conflict between random assignment and treatment preference: Implications for internal validity. *Evaluation and Program Planning, 26*(2), 109–121. https://doi.org/10.1016/S0149-7189(03)00014-4

Council for Accreditation of Counseling and Related Educational Programs. (2016). *Standards.* https://www.cacrep.org/for-programs/2016-cacrep-standards/

Council on Social Work Education. (2015). *Educational competencies.* www.bu.edu/ssw/files/2016/07/CSWE-2015-Competencies.pdf

Covey, S. R. (1990). *The 7 habits of highly effective people.* Fireside.

COVID-19 Hate Crimes Act (Pub. L. 117-13). (2021).

Cragun, C. L., & Friedlander, M. L. (2012). Experiences of Christian clients in secular psychotherapy: A mixed-methods investigation. *Journal of Counseling Psychology, 59*(3), 379–391. https://doi.org/10.1037/a0028283

Creaven, A.-M., Healy, A., & Howard, S. (2018). Social connectedness and depression: Is there added value in volunteering? *Journal of Social and Personal Relationships, 35*(10), 1400–1417. https://doi.org/10.1177/0265407517716786

Cross, W. E. (1971). The Negro-to-Black conversion experience. *Black World*, 20(9), 13–27.

Davis, D., DeBlaere, C., Hook, J., & Owen, J. (2020). *Mindfulness-based practices in therapy: A cultural humility approach*. American Psychological Association. https://doi.org/10.1037/0000156-000

Davis, D. E., DeBlaere, C., Owen, J., Hook, J. N., Rivera, D. P., Choe, E., Van Tongeren, D. R., Worthington, E. L., Jr., & Placeres, V. (2018). The multicultural orientation framework: A narrative review. *Psychotherapy: Theory, Research, & Practice*, 55(1), 89–100. https://doi.org/10.1037/pst0000160

Davis, D. E., Worthington, E. L., Jr., Hook, J. N., Emmons, R. A., Hill, P. C., Bollinger, R. A., & Van Tongeren, D. R. (2013). Humility and the development and repair of social bonds: Two longitudinal studies. *Self and Identity*, 12(1), 58–77. https://doi.org/10.1080/15298868.2011.636509

de las Fuentes, C. (2012). Working with men in the minority: Multiple identities, multiple selves. In H. Sweet (Ed.), *Gender in the therapy hour: Voices of women clinicians working with men* (pp. 149–170). Taylor and Francis.

de las Fuentes, C., Ramos Duffer, M., & Vasquez, M. J. T. (2013). Gendered borders: Forensic evaluations of immigrant women. *Women & Therapy*, 36(3–4), 302–318. https://doi.org/10.1080/02703149.2013.797782

DeAngelis, T. (2010). Found in translation. *Monitor on Psychology*, 41(2), 52–55. https://www.apa.org/monitor/2010/02/translation

Delgado, R. (2009). The law of the noose: A history of Latino lynching. *Harvard Civil Rights–Civil Liberties Law Review (CR-CL)*, 44 (U. of Alabama Legal Studies Research Paper 2533521). https://ssrn.com/sbstract=2533521

DeNisco, S. (2011). Exploring the relationship between resilience and diabetes outcomes in African Americans. *Journal of the American Academy of Nurse Practitioners*, 23(11), 602–610. https://doi.org/10.1111/j.1745-7599.2011.00648.x

Deutsch, J. I. (2019). The eugenics crusade. *The Journal of American History*, 106(1), 284–285. https://doi.org/10.1093/jahist/jaz330

Diana v. State Board of Education, CA 70 RFT (N.D. Cal. 1970).

Diaz-Martinez, A. M., Interian, A., & Waters, D. M. (2010). The integration of CBT, multicultural and feminist psychotherapies with Latinas. *Journal of Psychotherapy Integration*, 20(3), 312–326. https://doi.org/10.1037/a0020819

Dovidio, J. F., Gaertner, S. L., Kawakami, K., & Hodson, G. (2002). Why can't we just get along? Interpersonal biases and interracial distrust. *Cultural Diversity & Ethnic Minority Psychology*, 8(2), 88–102. https://doi.org/10.1037/1099-9809.8.2.88

Dovidio, J. F., Gaertner, S. L., & Pearson, A. R. (2016). Racism among the well-intentioned: Bias without awareness. In A. G. Miller (Ed.), *The social psychology of good and evil* (2nd ed., pp. 1–43). Guilford Press.

Eberhardt, J. L. (2005). Imaging race. *American Psychologist, 60*(2), 181–190. https://doi.org/10.1037/0003-066X.60.2.181

Ellis, A. (1980). *The case against religion: A psychotherapist's view and the case against religiosity.* American Atheist Press.

Executive Order No. 13769, 82 FR 8977 (2017).

Falender, C. A., & Shafranske, E. P. (2016). *Supervision essentials for the practice of competency-based supervision.* American Psychological Association. 10.1037/15962-000

Falender, C. A., Shafranske, E. P., & Falicov, C. (2014). Diversity and multiculturalism in supervision. In C. A. Falender, E. P. Shafranske, & C. Falicov (Eds.), *Multiculturalism and diversity in clinical supervision: A competency-based approach* (pp. 3–28). American Psychological Association. https://doi.org/10.1037/14370-001

Felder, A., & Robbins, B. (2016). The integrated heart of cultural and mindfulness meditation practice in existential phenomenology and humanistic psychotherapy. *The Humanistic Psychologist, 44*(2), 105–126. https://doi.org/10.1037/hum0000021

Felitti, V. J., Anda, R. F., Nordenberg, D., Williamson, D. F., Spitz, A. M., Edwards, V., Koss, M. P., & Marks, J. S. (1998). Relationship of childhood abuse and household dysfunction to many of the leading causes of death in adults. The Adverse Childhood Experiences (ACE) Study. *American Journal of Preventive Medicine, 14*(4), 245–258. https://doi.org/10.1016/S0749-3797(98)00017-8

Finn, J. L. (2020). *Just practice: A social justice approach to social work.* Oxford University Press.

Fischer, A. R., Jome, L. M., & Atkinson, D. R. (1998). Reconceptualizing multicultural counseling: Universal healing conditions in a culturally specific context. *The Counseling Psychologist, 26*(4), 525–588. https://doi.org/10.1177/0011000098264001

Flannagan, J. (2018, January 10). Person-centered spirituality. *Counseling and Psychotherapy Theory and Practice.* https://johnsommersflanagan.com/2018/01/10/person-centered-spirituality/

Fong, E., Ficklin, S., & Lee, H. (2017). Increasing cultural understanding and diversity in applied behavior analysis. *Behavior Analysis: Research and Practice, 17*(2), 103–113. https://doi.org/10.1037/bar0000076

Fouad, N. A., & Arredondo, P. (2007). *Becoming culturally oriented: Practical advice for psychologists and educators.* American Psychological Association. https://doi.org/10.1037/11483-000

Foxman, A. H., & Wolf, C. (2013). *Viral hate: Containing its spread on the internet.* Palgrave Macmillan. 10.1111/1478-9302.12087_70

Frank, J. D., & Frank, J. B. (1991). *Persuasion and healing: A comparative study of psychotherapy* (3rd ed.). Johns Hopkins University Press.

Franklin, A. J. (2009). Reflections on ethnic minority psychology: Learning from our past so the present informs our future. *Cultural Diversity & Ethnic Minority Psychology, 15*(4), 416–424. https://doi.org/10.1037/a0017560

Frey, J. R. (2019). Assessment for special education: Diagnosis and placement. *The Annals of the American Academy of Political and Social Science, 683*(1), 149–161. https://doi.org/10.1177/0002716219841352

Frosh, S. (2013). Psychoanalysis, colonialism, racism. *Journal of Theoretical and Philosophical Psychology, 33*(3), 141–154. https://doi.org/10.1037/a0033398

Fuertes, J. N., Brady-Amoon, P., Thind, N., & Chang, T. (2015). The therapy relationship in multicultural psychotherapy. *Psychotherapy Bulletin, 50*(1), 41–45.

Fuertes, J. N., Mueller, L. N., Chauhan, R. V., Walker, J. A., & Ladany, N. (2002). An investigation of European American therapists' approach to counseling African American clients. *The Counseling Psychologist, 30*(5), 763–788. https://doi.org/10.1177/0011000002305007

Gaertner, S. L., & Dovidio, J. F. (2000). *Reducing intergroup bias: The common ingroup identity model.* Brunner/Mazel. 10.4324/9781315804576

Gallup, G., & Lindsay, D. (1999). *Surveying the religious landscape: Trends in US beliefs.* Morehouse Publishing.

Gamboa, S. (2015, June 16). *Donald Trump announces a presidential bid by trashing Mexico, Mexicans.* NBC News. https://www.nbcnews.com/news/latino/donald-trump-announces-presidential-bid-trashing-mexico-mexicansn376521

Garcia, M. (2016). Racist in the machine: The disturbing implications of algorithmic bias. *World Policy Journal, 33*(4), 111–117.

Gaztambide, D. J. (2018). Review of psychoanalytic theory and cultural competence in psychotherapy [Review of the book *Psychoanalytic theory and cultural competence in psychotherapy*, by P. Tummala-Narra]. *Psychoanalytic Psychology, 35*(4), 468–472. https://doi.org/10.1037/pap0000174

Geller, S. E., Koch, A. R., Roesch, P., Filut, A., Hallgren, E., & Carnes, M. (2018). The more things change, the more they stay the same: A study to evaluate compliance with inclusion and assessment of women and minorities in randomized controlled trials. *Academic Medicine, 93*(4), 630–635. https://doi.org/10.1097/ACM.0000000000002027

Gibbons, M. B. C., Gallop, R., Thompson, D., Gaines, A., Rieger, A., & Crits-Christoph, P. (2019). Predictors of treatment attendance in cognitive and dynamic therapies for major depressive disorder delivered in a community mental health setting. *Journal of Consulting and Clinical Psychology, 87*(8), 745–755. https://doi.org/10.1037/ccp0000414

Gibbons, S. B. (2011). Understanding empathy as a complex construct: A review of the literature. *Clinical Social Work Journal, 39*(3), 243–252. https://doi.org/10.1007/s10615-010-0305-2

Gold, B. T., Kim, C., Johnson, N. F., Kryscio, R. J., & Smith, C. D. (2013). Lifelong bilingualism maintains neural efficiency for cognitive control in aging. *The Journal of Neuroscience, 33*(2), 387–396. https://doi.org/10.1523/JNEUROSCI.3837-12.2013

Gómez, J. M., Caño, A., & Baltes, B. B. (2021). Who are we missing? Examining the Graduate Record Examination quantitative score as a barrier to admission into psychology doctoral programs for capable ethnic minorities. *Training and Education in Professional Psychology, 15*(3), 211–218. https://doi.org/10.1037/tep0000336

Gonzalez, D. O., Suleiman, L. I., Ivey, G. D., & Callender, C. O. (2011). Is there a role for race in science and medicine. *Bulletin of the American College of Surgeons, 96*(9), 12–18.

Goode, T., & Jones, W. (2009). *Linguistic competence.* https://nccc.georgetown.edu/documents/Definition%20of%20Linguistic%20Competence.pdf

Goode-Cross, D. T., & Grim, K. A. (2016). "An unspoken level of comfort": Black therapists' experiences working with Black clients. *The Journal of Black Psychology, 42*(1), 29–53. https://doi.org/10.1177/0095798414552103

Goodell, R. (2020, June 5). *NFL condemns racism, apologizes for not listening to players earlier.* CBS Los Angeles. https://losangeles.cbslocal.com/2020/06/05/nfl-apologizes-roger-goodell-twitter-colin-kaepernick/

Goodwin, B. J., Coyne, A. E., & Constantino, M. J. (2018). Extending the context-responsive psychotherapy integration framework to cultural processes in psychotherapy. *Psychotherapy: Theory, Research, & Practice, 55*(1), 3–8. https://doi.org/10.1037/pst0000143

Gramlich, J. (2019, May 21). *From police to parole, Black and White Americans differ widely in their views of criminal justice system.* Pew Research Center. https://www.pewresearch.org/fact-tank/2019/05/21/from-police-to-parole-black-and-white-americans-differ-widely-in-their-views-of-criminal-justice-system/

Green, B. (2007, January). *The complexity of diversity: Multiple identities and the denial of privilege (within marginalized groups)* [Keynote address]. National Multicultural Conference and Summit, Seattle, WA, United States.

Greenwald, A. G., & Banaji, M. R. (1995). Implicit social cognition: Attitudes, self-esteem, and stereotypes. *Psychological Review, 102*(1), 4–27. https://doi.org/10.1037/0033-295X.102.1.4

Grindal, T., Schifter, L., Schwartz, G., & Hehir, T. (2019). Racial differences in special education identification and placement: Evidence across three states.

Harvard Educational Review, 89(4), 525–553. https://doi.org/10.17763/1943-5045-89.4.525

Guidi, J., Lucente, M., Sonino, N., & Fava, G. A. (2021). Allostatic load and its impact on health: A systematic review. *Psychotherapy and Psychosomatics, 90*(1), 11–27. https://doi.org/10.1159/000510696

Guthrie, R. V. (1976). *Even the rat was white: A historical view of psychology.* Harper & Row. 10.1002/1520-6696(197804)14:2<181:AID-JHBS2300140212>3.0.CO;2-D

Guthrie, R. V. (1998). *Even the rat was white: A historical view of psychology* (2nd ed.). Allyn & Bacon.

Hall, G. C. N., Yip, T., & Zárate, M. A. (2016). On becoming multicultural in a monocultural research world: A conceptual approach to studying ethnocultural diversity. *American Psychologist, 71*(1), 40–51. https://doi.org/10.1037/a0039734

Hartelius, G., Caplan, M., & Rardin, M. A. (2007). Transpersonal psychology: Defining the past, divining the future. *The Humanistic Psychologist, 35*(2), 135–160. https://doi.org/10.1080/08873260701274017

Hayes, J. A., McAleavey, A. A., Castonguay, L. G., & Locke, B. D. (2016). Psychotherapists' outcomes with White and racial/ethnic minority clients: First, the good news. *Journal of Counseling Psychology, 63*(3), 261–268. https://doi.org/10.1037/cou0000098

Hayes-Bautista, D. (1992). *No longer a minority: Latinos and social policy in California.* University of California, Los Angeles, Chicano Studies Research Center.

Hays, D. G., Arredondo, P., Gladding, S. T., & Toporek, R. L. (2010). Integrating social justice in group work: The next decade. *Journal for Specialists in Group Work, 35*(2), 177–206. https://doi.org/10.1080/01933921003706022

Hays, P. A. (2009). Integrating evidence-based practice, cognitive-behavior therapy, and multicultural therapy: Ten steps for culturally competent practice. *Professional Psychology: Research and Practice, 40*(4), 354–360. https://doi.org/10.1037/a0016250

Hays, P. A. (2016). *Addressing cultural complexities in practice: Assessment, diagnosis, and therapy* (3rd ed.). American Psychological Association. https://doi.org/10.1037/14801-000

Hays, P. A. (2019). Introduction. In G. Y. Iwamasa & P. A. Hays (Eds.), *Culturally responsive cognitive behavioral therapy: Practice and supervision* (2nd ed., pp. 3–24). https://doi.org/10.1037/0000119-001

Helms, J. E., Jernigan, M., & Mascher, J. (2005). The meaning of race in psychology and how to change it: A methodological perspective. *American Psychologist, 60*(1), 27–36. https://doi.org/10.1037/0003-066X.60.1.27

Hewstone, M., Rubin, M., & Willis, H. (2002). Intergroup bias. *Annual Review of Psychology, 53*(1), 575–604. https://doi.org/10.1146/annurev.psych.53.100901.135109

Hill, C. E., Thompson, B. J., Cogar, M. C., & Denman, D. W. (1993). Beneath the surface of long-term therapy: Therapist and client report of their own and each other's covert processes. *Journal of Counseling Psychology, 40*(3), 278–287. https://doi.org/10.1037/0022-0167.40.3.278

Hill, C. E., & Williams, E. N. (2000). The process of individual therapy. In S. D. Brown & R. W. Lent (Eds.), *Handbook of counseling psychology* (pp. 670–710). Wiley.

Hillenbrand, L. (2010). *Unbroken: A World War II story of survival, resilience, and redemption.* Random House.

Ho, M. K., & McDowell, E. (1973). The Black worker–White client relationship. *Clinical Social Work Journal, 1*(3), 161–167. https://doi.org/10.1007/BF01786037

Hoffman, L., Cleare-Hoffman, H., & Jackson, T. (2015). Humanistic psychology and multiculturalism: History, current status, and advancements. In K. J. Schneider, J. F. Pierson, & J. F. T. Bugental (Eds.), *The handbook of humanistic psychology: Theory, research, and practice* (pp. 41–56). SAGE Publications. https://doi.org/10.4135/9781483387864.n4

Hofstra, B., Kulkarni, V. V., Munoz-Najar Galvez, S., He, B., Jurafsky, D., & McFarland, D. A. (2020). The diversity-innovation paradox in science. *Proceedings of the National Academy of Sciences, 117*(17), 9284–9291. https://doi.org/10.1073/pnas.1915378117

Holkup, P. A., Tripp-Reimer, T., Salois, E. M., & Weinert, C. (2004). Community-based participatory research: An approach to intervention research with a Native American community. *Advances in Nursing Science, 27*(3), 162–175. https://doi.org/10.1097/00012272-200407000-00002

Holliday, B. G. (2009). The history and visions of African American psychology: Multiple pathways to place, space, and authority. *Cultural Diversity & Ethnic Minority Psychology, 15*(4), 317–337. https://doi.org/10.1037/a0016971

Holliday, B. G., & Holmes, A. L. (2003). A tale of challenge and change: A history and chronology of ethnic minorities in psychology in the United States. In G. Bernal, J. E. Trimble, A. K. Burlew, & F. T. L. Leong (Eds.), *Handbook of racial and ethnic minority psychology* (pp. 15–64). Sage. https://doi.org/10.4135/9781412976008.n2

Hook, J. N., Davis, D. E., Owen, J., Worthington, E. L., Jr., & Utsey, S. O. (2013). Cultural humility: Measuring openness to culturally diverse clients. *Journal of Counseling Psychology, 60*(3), 353–366. https://doi.org/10.1037/a0032595

Hook, J. N., Davis, D. E., Van Tongeren, D. R., Hill, P. C., Worthington, E. L., Jr., Farrell, J. E., & Dieke, P. (2015). Intellectual humility and forgiveness of religious leaders. *The Journal of Positive Psychology, 10*(6), 499–506. https://doi.org/10.1080/17439760.2015.1004554

Hook, J. N., Watkins, C. E., Jr., Davis, D. E., Owen, J., Van Tongeren, D. R., & Ramos, M. J. (2016). Cultural humility in psychotherapy supervision. *American Journal of Psychotherapy, 70*(2), 149–166. https://doi.org/10.1176/appi.psychotherapy.2016.70.2.149

Hoover, S. M. (2016). A critical feminist phenomenological study of social justice identity among professional psychologists and trainees from a feminist multicultural practicum. *Professional Psychology: Research and Practice, 47*(6), 383–390. https://doi.org/10.1037/pro0000110

How George Floyd's death reverberates around the world. (2020, June 8). In *The Economist.* https://www.economist.com/international/2020/06/08/how-george-floyds-death-reverberates-around-the-world

Huey, S. J., Jr., Tilley, J. L., Jones, E. O., & Smith, C. A. (2014). The contribution of cultural competence to evidence-based care for ethnically diverse populations. *Annual Review of Clinical Psychology, 10*(1), 305–338. https://doi.org/10.1146/annurev-clinpsy-032813-153729

Hughes, D. L., & DuMont, K. (2002). Using focus groups to facilitate culturally anchored research. In T. A. Revenson, A. R. D'Augelli, S. French, D. L. Hughes, D. Livert, E. Seidman, & H. Yoshikwawa (Eds.), *Ecological research to promote social change: Methodological advances from community psychology* (pp. 257–289). Kluwer Academic/Plenum Press Publishers. https://doi.org/10.1007/978-1-4615-0565-5_11

Hurtado, A. (2010). Multiple lenses: Multicultural feminist theory. In H. Landrine & N. F. Russo (Eds.), *Handbook of diversity of feminist psychology* (pp. 29–54). Springer.

Irby, B. J. (2013). *The handbook of educational theories.* Information Age Publishing.

Jamieson, J. P., Koslov, K., Nock, M. K., & Mendes, W. B. (2013). Experiencing discrimination increases risk taking. *Psychological Science, 24*(2), 131–139. https://doi.org/10.1177/0956797612448194

Johnson, R. N. (2008). *The psychology of racism: How internalized racism, academic self-concept, and campus racial climate impact the academic experiences and achievement of African American undergraduates* [Unpublished doctoral dissertation]. UCLA.

Jones, C. P. (2015). *All lives matter: Psychology's role in addressing the intersection of law enforcement practices and police-perpetrated violence in communities of color* [Panel presentation]. National Multicultural Conference and Summit. Atlanta, GA, United States.

Jones, J. M. (1998). Psychological knowledge and the new American dilemma of race. *Journal of Social Issues, 54*(4), 641–662. https://doi.org/10.1111/j.1540-4560.1998.tb01241.x

Kagawa-Singer, M., Dressler, W. W., George, S. M., & Ellwood, W. N. (2015). *The cultural framework for health: An integrative approach for research and program design and evaluation.* https://www.researchgate.net/profile/William-Elwood/publication/273970021_The_cultural_framework_for_health_An_integrative_approach_for_research_and_program_design_and_evaluation/links/5552200a08ae6943a86d6d4f/The-cultural-framework-for-health-An-integrative-approach-for-research-and-program-design-and-evaluation.pdf

Katsnelson, A. (2015). News feature: The neuroscience of poverty. *Proceedings of the National Academy of Sciences, 112*(51), 15530–15532. https://doi.org/10.1073/pnas.1522683112

Kelly, S., Bhagwat, R., Maynigo, P., & Moses, E. (2014). Couple and marital therapy: The complement and expansion provided by multicultural approaches. In F. T. L. Leong, L. Comas-Díaz, G. C. Nagayama Hall, V. C. McLoyd, & J. E. Trimble (Eds.), *APA handbook of multicultural psychology: Vol. 2. Applications and training* (pp. 479–497). American Psychological Association. https://doi.org/10.1037/14187-027

Killian, T., Cardona, B., & Hudspeth, E. (2017). Culturally responsive play therapy with Somali refugees. *International Journal of Play Therapy, 26*(1), 23–32. https://doi.org/10.1037/pla0000040

Kilmer, E. D., Villarreal, C., Janis, B. M., Callahan, J. L., Ruggero, C. J., Kilmer, J. N., Love, P. K., & Cox, R. J. (2019). Differential early termination is tied to client race/ethnicity status. *Practice Innovations, 4*(2), 88–98. https://doi.org/10.1037/pri0000085

King, B. R., & Boswell, J. F. (2019). Therapeutic strategies and techniques in early cognitive-behavioral therapy. *Psychotherapy: Theory, Research, & Practice, 56*(1), 35–40. https://doi.org/10.1037/pst0000202

King-Spooner, S. (2001). The place of spirituality in psychotherapy. In S. King-Spooner & C. Newnes (Eds.), *Spirituality and psychotherapy* (pp. 28–36). PCCS Books.

Kivlighan, D. M., III, & Chapman, N. A. (2018). Extending the multicultural orientation (MCO) framework to group psychotherapy: A clinical illustration. *Psychotherapy, 55*(1), 39–44. https://doi.org/10.1037/pst0000142

Kivlighan, D. M., III, Swancy, A. G., Smith, E., & Brennaman, C. (2021). Examining racial microaggressions in group therapy and the buffering role of members' perceptions of their group's multicultural orientation. *Journal of Counseling Psychology, 68*(5), 621–628. https://doi.org/10.1037/cou0000531

Kleinman, A. (1988). *The illness narratives: Suffering, healing and the human condition.* Basic Books. 10.1177/136346158902600303

Knowles, E. D., Lowery, B. S., Hogan, C. M., & Chow, R. M. (2009). On the malleability of ideology: Motivated construals of color blindness. *Journal of Personality and Social Psychology, 96*(4), 857–869. https://doi.org/10.1037/a0013595

Koç, V., & Kafa, G. (2019). Cross-cultural research on psychotherapy: The need for a change. *Journal of Cross-Cultural Psychology, 50*(1), 100–115. https://doi.org/10.1177/0022022118806577

Krause, N., & Chatters, L. M. (2005). Exploring race differences in a Multi-dimensional Battery of Prayer Measures among older adults. *Sociology of Religion, 66*(1), 23–43. https://doi.org/10.2307/4153114

Kristof, N. (2020, June 28). Learning from Hispanic Americans. *The New York Times, SR*, p. 9.

Kugelmass, H. (2016). "Sorry, I'm not accepting new patients": An audit study of access to mental health care. *Journal of Health and Social Behavior, 57*(2), 168–183. https://doi.org/10.1177/0022146516647098

Kuo, B. C. H. (2021, April 16th). *Foundations of cultural competence, cultural humility, & culturally-informed practice: An introduction* [Conference workshop]. Michigan Psychological Association Spring Annual Conference.

La Roche, M. J. (2013). *Cultural psychotherapy: Theory, methods, and practice.* Sage Publications.

La Roche, M. J. (2021). Changing multicultural guidelines: Clinical and research implications for evidence-based psychotherapies. *Professional Psychology: Research and Practice, 52*(2), 111–120. https://doi.org/10.1037/pro0000347

Lambert, M. J. (2013). The efficacy and effectiveness of psychotherapy. In M. J. Lambert (Ed.), *Bergin and Garfield's handbook of psychotherapy and behavior change* (6th ed., pp. 169–218). John Wiley & Sons.

Lancaster, C., Dominguez, D., Lopez, S., Garcia, R., & Constantin, D. (2015). Enacting social justice through the advocacy competencies. *Vistas Online Article, 61*. https://www.counseling.org/docs/default-source/vistas/article_617d5a22f16116603abcacff0000bee5e7.pdf?sfvrsn=e34c422c_4

Larry P. v. Riles, 495 F. Supp. 926 (N.D. Cal. 1979).

Lattuada, P. L. (2018). Transpersonal psychology as a science. *Integral Transpersonal Journal, 11*(11), 26–51. https://doi.org/10.32031/ITIBTE_ITJ_11-LP2

Lau, A. S., Chang, D. F., & Okazaki, S. (2010). Methodological challenges in treatment outcome research with ethnic minorities. *Cultural Diversity & Ethnic Minority Psychology, 16*(4), 573–580. https://doi.org/10.1037/a0021371

Leong, F. T. L. (2009). Guest editor's introduction: History of racial and ethnic minority psychology. *Cultural Diversity & Ethnic Minority Psychology, 15*(4), 315–316. https://doi.org/10.1037/a0017556

Leong, F. T. L., & Kalibatseva, Z. (2016). Threats to cultural validity in clinical diagnosis and assessment: Illustrated with the case of Asian Americans. In N. Zane, G. Bernal, & F. T. L. Leong (Eds.), *Evidence-based psychological practice with ethnic minorities: Culturally informed research and clinical strategies* (pp. 57–74). American Psychological Association. https://doi.org/10.1037/14940-004

Leong, F. T. L., Lui, P. P., & Kalibatseva, Z. (2020). Multicultural issues in clinical psychological assessment. In M. Sellbom & J. A. Suhr (Eds.), *The Cambridge handbook of clinical assessment and diagnosis* (pp. 25–37). Cambridge University Press.

Leong, F. T. L., & Okazaki, S. (2009). History of Asian American psychology. *Cultural Diversity & Ethnic Minority Psychology, 15*(4), 352–362. https://doi.org/10.1037/a0016443

Leong, F. T. L., Pickren, W. E., & Vasquez, M. J. T. (2017). APA efforts in promoting human rights and social justice. *American Psychologist, 72*(8), 778–790. https://doi.org/10.1037/amp0000220

Levin, J. S., Taylor, R. J., & Chatters, L. M. (1994). Race and gender differences in religiosity among older adults: Findings from four national surveys. *Journal of Gerontology, 49*(3), S137–S145. https://doi.org/10.1093/geronj/49.3.S137

Lonner, W. J., Draguns, J. G., Trimble, J. E., & Scharron-del Rio, M. R. (2016). Dedication: Our deepest thanks to Paul B. Pedersen—Friend, scholar and gentleman. In P. B. Pedersen, W. J. Lonner, J. G. Draguns, J. E. Trimble, & M. R. Scharron-del Rio (Eds.), *Counseling across cultures* (7th ed., pp. xvii–xx). Sage.

Love, M., Smith, A., Lyall, S., Mullins, J., & Cohn, T. (2015). Exploring the relationship between gay affirmative practice and empathy among mental health professionals. *Journal of Multicultural Counseling and Development, 43*(2), 83–96. https://doi.org/10.1002/j.2161-1912.2015.00066.x

Lowe, S. M., & Mascher, J. (2001). The role of sexual orientation in multicultural counseling: Integrating bodies of knowledge. In J. G. Ponterotto, J. M. Casas, L. A. Suzuki, & C. M. Alexander (Eds.), *Handbook of multicultural counseling* (pp. 755–778). Sage Publications.

Lum, K., & Johndrow, J. E. (2016). *A statistical framework for fair predictive algorithms.* arXiv:1610.08077

Mahalingam, R. (2007). Essentialism, power and the representation of social categories: An integrated perspective. *Human Development, 50*(6), 300–319. https://doi.org/10.1159/000109832

Manning, L. K. (2013). Navigating hardships in old age: Exploring the relationship between spirituality and resilience in later life. *Qualitative Health Research, 23*(4), 568–575. https://doi.org/10.1177/1049732312471730

Marsella, A., & Pedersen, P. (1980). *Cross-cultural counseling and psychotherapy: Foundations, evaluation, ethnocultural considerations, and future perspectives.* Pergamon.

Maschi, T., Baer, J., & Turner, S. (2011). The psychological goods on clinical social work: A content analysis of the clinical social work and social justice literature. *Journal of Social Work Practice, 25*(2), 233–253. https://doi.org/10.1080/02650533.2010.544847

Matthew Shepard and James Byrd Jr., Hate Crimes Prevention Act, Public Law Number 111–84 (2009).

McCubbin, L. D., & Marsella, A. (2009). Native Hawaiians and psychology: The cultural and historical context of indigenous ways of knowing. *Cultural Diversity & Ethnic Minority Psychology, 15*(4), 374–387. https://doi.org/10.1037/a0016774

McEwen, B. S., & Stellar, E. (1993). Stress and the individual. Mechanisms leading to disease. *Archives of Internal Medicine, 153*(18), 2093–2101. https://doi.org/10.1001/archinte.1993.00410180039004

McGhee, H. (2021). *The sum of us: What racism costs everyone and how we can prosper together.* Random House.

McGoldrick, M., Giordano, J., & Garcia-Prieto, N. (2005). Overview: Ethnicity and family therapy. In M. McGoldrick, J. Giordano, & J. Pearce (Eds.), *Ethnicity & family therapy* (3rd ed., pp. 1–40). Guilford Press.

McGuire, T. G., & Miranda, J. (2008). New evidence regarding racial and ethnic disparities in mental health care: Policy implications. *Health Affairs, 27*(2). https://doi.org/10.1377/hlthaff.27.2.393

McIntosh, P. (1988). *White privilege and male privilege: A personal account of coming to see correspondences through work in women's studies* (Working Paper 189). Center for Research on Women. https://www.wcwonline.org/images/pdf/White_Privilege_and_Male_Privilege_Personal_Account-Peggy_McIntosh.pdf

Medin, D., & Lee, C. (2012, May/June). Diversity makes better science. *Observer.* https://www.psychologicalscience.org/observer/diversity-makes-better-science

Melville, M. B. (1980). *Twice a minority: Mexican American women.* Mosby.

Mendes, W. B., Gray, H. M., Mendoza-Denton, R., Major, B., & Epel, E. S. (2007). Why egalitarianism might be good for your health: Physiological thriving during stressful intergroup encounters. *Psychological Science, 18*(11), 991–998. https://doi.org/10.1111/j.1467-9280.2007.02014.x

Merrick, M. T., & Guinn, A. S. (2018). Child abuse and neglect: Breaking the intergenerational link. *American Journal of Public Health, 108*(9), 1117–1118. https://doi.org/10.2105/AJPH.2018.304636

Metzler, M., Merrick, M. T., Klevens, J., Ports, K. A., & Ford, D. C. (2017). Adverse childhood experiences and life opportunities: Shifting the narrative. *Children and Youth Services Review, 72*, 141–149. https://doi.org/10.1016/j.childyouth.2016.10.021

Meyers, S. (2007, October 1). Putting social justice into practice in psychology courses. *Observer.* https://www.psychologicalscience.org/observer/putting-social-justice-into-practice-in-psychology-courses

Michael, A., & Bartoli, E. (2017). Comprehensive multicultural counseling curriculum: Self-awareness as process. In R. Allan & S. S. Poulsen (Eds.), *Creating cultural safety in couples and family therapy: Supervision and training* (pp. 71–87). Springer International Publishing AG. https://doi.org/10.1007/978-3-319-64617-6_7

Michel, A. (2018, July 13). The paradox of diversity. *Observer.* https://www.psychologicalscience.org/observer/the-paradox-of-diversity

Miles, J. R., Anders, C., Kivlighan, D. M., III, & Belcher Platt, A. A. (2021). Cultural ruptures: Addressing microaggressions in group therapy. *Group Dynamics: Theory, Research, and Practice, 25*(1), 74–88. https://doi.org/10.1037/gdn0000149

Miles, J. R., & Paquin, J. D. (2014, August 7–10). *Teaching at the intersection of evidence-based practice and multicultural competence in group training* [Symposium]. American Psychological Association 122nd Annual Convention, Washington, DC, United States.

Millett, G. A., Jones, A. T., Benkeser, D., Baral, S., Mercer, L., Beyrer, C., Honermann, B., Lankiewicz, E., Mena, L., Crowley, J. S., Sherwood, J., & Sullivan, P. S. (2020). Assessing differential impacts of COVID-19 on Black communities. *Annals of Epidemiology, 47*, 37–44. https://doi.org/10.1016/j.annepidem.2020.05.003

Milne, D. L., & Watkins, C. E., Jr. (2014). Defining and understanding clinical supervision: A functional approach. In C. E. Watkins Jr. & D. L. Milne (Eds.), *The Wiley international handbook of clinical supervision* (pp. 1–19). Wiley. https://doi.org/10.1002/9781118846360.ch1

Mio, J. S. (2003). On teaching multiculturalism: History, models, and content. In G. Bernal, J. E. Trimble, A. K. Burlew, & F. T. L. Leong (Eds.), *Handbook of ethnic and racial minority psychology* (pp. 119–146). Sage. https://doi.org/10.4135/9781412976008.n6

Mio, J. S., Barker-Hackett, L., & Tumambing, J. S. (2006). *Multicultural psychology: Understanding our diverse communities.* McGraw Hill.

Mio, J. S., Barker-Hackett, L., & Tumambing, J. S. (2009). *Multicultural psychology: Understanding our diverse communities* (2nd ed.). McGraw-Hill.

Miranda, J., Green, B. L., Krupnick, J. L., Chung, J., Siddique, J., Belin, T., & Revicki, D. (2006). One-year outcomes of a randomized clinical trial treating depression in low-income minority women. *Journal of Consulting and Clinical Psychology, 74*(1), 99–111. https://doi.org/10.1037/0022-006X.74.1.99

Mishne, J. M. (2002). *Multiculturalism and the therapeutic process.* Guilford Press.

Moodley, R., & Palmer, S. (Eds.). (2014). *Race, culture and psychotherapy: Critical perspectives in multicultural practice.* Routledge. 10.4324/9781315820194

Mosher, D. K., Hook, J. N., Captari, L. E., Davis, D. E., DeBlaere, C., & Owen, J. (2017). Cultural humility: A therapeutic framework for engaging diverse clients. *Practice Innovations, 2*(4), 221–233. https://doi.org/10.1037/pri0000055

Motulsky, S. L., Gere, S. H., Saleem, R., & Trantham, S. M. (2014). Teaching social justice counseling psychology. *The Counseling Psychologist, 42*(8), 1058–1083. https://doi.org/10.1177/0011000014553855

Muñoz, R. F., & Mendelson, T. (2005). Toward evidence-based interventions for diverse populations: The San Francisco General Hospital prevention and treatment manuals. *Journal of Consulting and Clinical Psychology, 73*(5), 790–799. https://doi.org/10.1037/0022-006X.73.5.790

National Association of School Psychologists. (2020). *The professional standards.* https://www.nasponline.org/standards-and-certification/nasp-2020-professional-standards-adopted

National Association of Social Workers. (2015). *Standards and indicators for cultural competence in social work practice.* https://www.socialworkers.org/LinkClick.aspx?fileticket=7dVckZAYUmk%3D&portalid=0

National Center for Cultural Competence. (2004). *Bridging the cultural divide in healthcare settings: The essential role of health care broker programs.* https://nccc.georgetown.edu/documents/Cultural_Broker_Guide_English.pdf

National Institute of Mental Health. (2017a). *Collaborative hubs to reduce the burden of suicide among American Indian and Alaska Native youth.* https://www.nimh.nih.gov/about/organization/od/odwd/ai-an/index.shtml

National Institute of Mental Health. (2017b). *Mental illness.* https://www.nimh.nih.gov/health/statistics/mental-illness.shtml

National Institute of Mental Health. (2017c). *Suicide.* https://www.nimh.nih.gov/health/statistics/suicide.shtml

National Institute on Minority Health and Health Disparities (NIMHD), National Institute of Mental Health. (2015, August 26). *Cross-cutting aspects of the NIMH strategic plan for research* [Webinar]. https://www.nimh.nih.gov/news/

events/2015/mental-health-disparities-research-at-the-national-institute-of-mental-health-nimh-cross-cutting-aspects-of-the-nimh-strategic-plan-for-research.html

National Institute on Minority Health and Health Disparities (NIMHD), National Institute of Mental Health. (2020). *The NIH almanac.* https://www.nih.gov/about-nih/what-we-do/nih-almanac/national-institute-minority-health-health-disparities-nimhd

National Institutes of Health. (2001). *NIH policy and guidelines on the inclusion of women and minorities as subjects in clinical research.* https://grants.nih.gov/policy/inclusion/women-and-minorities/guidelines.htm

National Institutes of Health. (2017, February 15). Cultural respect. *Clear communication.* https://www.nih.gov/institutes-nih/nih-office-director/office-communications-public-liaison/clear-communication/cultural-respect

National Institutes of Health. (2018). *Guidance for reporting valid analysis as required by the NIH policy and guidelines on the inclusion of women and minorities as subjects in clinical research* (NOT-OD-18-014). https://grants.nih.gov/sites/default/files/Valid%20analysis%20CTgov%20guidance%20final_508c.pdf

Nelson, D. W., & Baumgarte, R. (2004). Cross-cultural misunderstandings reduce empathic responding. *Journal of Applied Social Psychology, 34*(2), 391–401. https://doi.org/10.1111/j.1559-1816.2004.tb02553.x

Norcross, J. C. (1990). An eclectic definition of psychotherapy. In J. K. Zeig & W. M. Munion (Eds.), *What is psychotherapy? Contemporary perspectives* (pp. 218–220). Jossey-Bass.

Norcross, J. C., Hedges, M., & Prochaska, J. O. (2002). The face of 2010: A Delphi poll on the future of psychotherapy. *Professional Psychology: Research and Practice, 33*(3), 316–322. https://doi.org/10.1037/0735-7028.33.3.316

Norcross, J. C., & Lambert, M. J. (2011). Evidence-based therapy relationships. In J. C. Norcross (Ed.), *Psychotherapy relationships that work: Evidence-based responsiveness* (2nd ed., pp. 3–22). Oxford University Press. https://doi.org/10.1093/acprof:oso/9780199737208.003.0001

Norcross, J. C., Pfund, R. A., & Prochaska, J. O. (2013). Psychotherapy in 2022: A Delphi poll on its future. *Professional Psychology: Research and Practice, 44*(5), 363–370. https://doi.org/10.1037/a0034633

Novacek, D. M., Hampton-Anderson, J. N., Ebor, M. T., Loeb, T. B., & Wyatt, G. E. (2020). Mental health ramifications of the COVID-19 pandemic for Black Americans: Clinical and research recommendations. *Psychological Trauma: Theory, Research, Practice, and Policy, 12*(5), 449–451. https://doi.org/10.1037/tra0000796

Occupational Therapy Professional Alliance of Canada. (2014). *Position statement: Diversity.* https://www.acotup-acpue.ca/english/documents/jointposition-statementondiversityfinalrevision25march2014.doc

Okazaki, S., David, E., & Abelmann, N. (2008). Colonialism and psychology of culture. *Social and Personality Psychology Compass, 2*(1), 90–106. https://doi.org/10.1111/j.1751-9004.2007.00046.x

Olver, K. (2012). Multicultural couples: Seeing the world through different lenses. In P. A. Robey, R. E. Wubbolding, & J. Carlson (Eds.), *Contemporary issues in couples counseling: A choice theory and reality therapy approach* (pp. 33–46). Routledge/Taylor & Francis Group.

Opotow, S. (1990). Moral exclusion and injustice: An introduction. *Journal of Social Issues, 46*(1), 1–20. https://doi.org/10.1111/j.1540-4560.1990.tb00268.x

Owen, J. (2013). Early career perspectives on psychotherapy research and practice: Psychotherapist effects, multicultural orientation, and couple interventions. *Psychotherapy: Theory, Research, & Practice, 50*(4), 496–502. https://doi.org/10.1037/a0034617

Owen, J., Leach, M. M., Wampold, B., & Rodolfa, E. (2011). Client and therapist variability in clients' perceptions of their therapists' multicultural competencies. *Journal of Counseling Psychology, 58*(1), 1–9. https://doi.org/10.1037/a0021496

Oxhandler, H. K., & Pargament, K. I. (2018). Measuring religious and spiritual competence across helping professions: Previous efforts and future directions. *Spirituality in Clinical Practice, 5*(2), 120–132. https://doi.org/10.1037/scp0000149

Pacheco, I., & Stamm, S. (2020, June 5). What CEOs said about George Floyd's death. *The Wall Street Journal.* https://www.wsj.com/articles/what-executives-said-about-george-floyds-death-11591364538?mod=hp_lead_pos10

Padilla, A. M., & Olmedo, E. (2009). Synopsis of key persons, events, and associations in the history of Latino psychology. *Cultural Diversity & Ethnic Minority Psychology, 15*(4), 363–373. https://doi.org/10.1037/a0017557

Palloni, A., & Morenoff, J. D. (2001). Interpreting the paradoxical in the Hispanic paradox: Demographic and epidemiologic approaches. *Annals of the New York Academy of Sciences, 954*(1), 140–174. https://doi.org/10.1111/j.1749-6632.2001.tb02751.x

Paniagua, F. A. (2018). ICD-10 versus *DSM-5* on cultural issues. *SAGE Open, 8*(1). Advance online publication. https://doi.org/10.1177/2158244018756165

Paquin, J. D., Tao, K. W., & Budge, S. L. (2019). Toward a psychotherapy science for all: Conducting ethical and socially just research. *Psychotherapy: Theory, Research, & Practice, 56*(4), 491–502. https://doi.org/10.1037/pst0000271

Pargament, K., & Cummings, J. (2010). Anchored by faith-religion as a resilience factor. In J. W. Reich, A. J. Zautra, & J. S. Hall (Eds.), *Handbook of adult resilience* (pp. 193–210). Guilford Press.

Patterson, C. H. (1989). Values in counseling and psychotherapy. *Counseling and Values*, *33*(3), 164–176. https://doi.org/10.1002/j.2161-007X.1989.tb00758.x

Pedersen, P. B. (Ed.). (1999a). *Multiculturalism as a fourth force*. Brunner/Mazel.

Pedersen, P. B. (1999b). Preface. In P. B. Pedersen (Ed.), *Multiculturalism as a fourth force* (pp. xxi–xxiii). Taylor & Francis.

Pedersen, P. B. (2002). The making of a culturally competent counselor. *Online Readings in Psychology and Culture*, *10*(3). Advance online publication. https://doi.org/10.9707/2307-0919.1093

Pedersen, P. B., Draguns, J. G., Lonner, W. J., & Trimble, J. E. (Eds.). (2002). Introduction: Multicultural awareness as a generic competence for counseling. In P. B. Pedersen, J. G. Draguns, W. J. Lonner, & J. E. Trimble (Eds.), *Counseling across cultures* (5th ed., pp. xii–xix). Sage.

Pedersen, P. B., Lonner, W. J., Draguns, J. G., Trimble, J. E., & Scharron-del Rio, M. R. (Eds.). (2016). *Counseling across cultures* (7th ed.). SAGE Publications. https://doi.org/10.4135/9781483398921

Pérez-Gualdrón, L. M., & Yeh, C. J. (2014). *Multicultural counseling and therapy counseling for social justice*. Oxford Handbooks Online. https://doi.org/10.1093/oxfordhb/9780199796694.013.020

Peters, H. C. (2017). Multicultural complexity: An intersectional lens for clinical supervision. *International Journal for the Advancement of Counseling*, *39*(2), 176–187. https://doi.org/10.1007/s10447-017-9290-2

Peterson, C., & Seligman, M. E. P. (2004). *Character strengths and virtues: A handbook and classification*. American Psychological Association; Oxford University Press.

Pettigrew, T. F., & Tropp, L. R. (2008). How does intergroup contact reduce prejudice? Meta-analytic test of three mediators. *European Journal of Social Psychology*, *38*(6), 922–934. https://doi.org/10.1002/ejsp.504

Philips, B., Karlsson, R., Nygren, R., Rother-Schirren, A., & Werbart, A. (2018). Early therapeutic process related to dropout in mentalization-based treatment with dual diagnosis patients. *Psychoanalytic Psychology*, *35*(2), 205–216. https://doi.org/10.1037/pap0000170

Phillips, J. C., Parent, M. C., Dozier, V. C., & Jackson, P. L. (2017). Depth of discussion of multicultural identities in supervision and supervisory outcomes. *Counselling Psychology Quarterly*, *30*(2), 188–210. https://doi.org/10.1080/09515070.2016.1169995

Phillips, N. L., Adams, G., & Salter, P. (2015). Beyond adaptation: Decolonizing approaches to coping with oppression. *Journal of Social and Political Psychology*, *3*(1), 365–387. https://doi.org/10.5964/jspp.v3i1.310

Plant, E. A., & Sachs-Ericsson, N. (2004). Racial and ethnic differences in depression: The roles of social support and meeting basic needs. *Journal of Consulting and Clinical Psychology, 72*(1), 41–52. https://doi.org/10.1037/0022-006X.72.1.41

Polo, A. J., Makol, B. A., Castro, A. S., Colón-Quintana, N., Wagstaff, A. E., & Guo, S. (2019). Diversity in randomized clinical trials of depression: A 36-year review. *Clinical Psychology Review, 67*, 22–35. https://doi.org/10.1016/j.cpr.2018.09.004

Poortinga, Y. H. (1999). Do differences in behaviour imply a need for different psychologies? *Applied Psychology, 48*(4), 419–432. https://doi.org/10.1080/026999499377394

Pope, K. S., & Vasquez, M. J. T. (1998). *Ethics in psychotherapy and counseling: A practical guide.* Jossey-Bass. 10.1080/00029157.2001.10403473

Pope, K. S., & Vasquez, M. J. T. (2016). *Ethics in psychotherapy and counseling: A practical guide* (5th ed.). John Wiley & Sons.

Pope, K. S., Vasquez, M. J. T., Chavez-Dueñas, N. Y., & Adames, H. Y. (2021). *Ethics in psychotherapy and counseling: A practical guide* (6th ed.). Wiley.

Porter, N. (1995). Supervision of psychotherapists: Integrating anti-racist, feminist, and multicultural perspectives. In H. Landrine (Ed.), *Bringing cultural diversity to feminist psychology: Theory, research, and practice* (pp. 163–175). American Psychological Association. https://doi.org/10.1037/10501-008

Price, J. H., & Khubchandani, J. (2017). Adolescent homicides, suicides, and the role of firearms: A narrative review. *Journal of Health Education, 48*(2), 67–79. https://doi.org/10.1080/19325037.2016.1272507

Purdie-Vaughns, V., Steele, C. M., Davies, P. G., Ditlmann, R., & Crosby, J. R. (2008). Social identity contingencies: How diversity cues signal threat or safety for African Americans in mainstream institutions. *Journal of Personality and Social Psychology, 94*(4), 615–630. https://doi.org/10.1037/0022-3514.94.4.615

Quinn, L. (2011, Spring). Working with interpreters in therapy. *Contemporary Psychotherapy, 3*(1). http://www.contemporarypsychotherapy.org/vol-3-no1-spring-2011/working-with-interpreters-in-therapy/

Ratts, M. J., & Pedersen, P. B. (2014). *Counseling for multiculturalism and social justice: Integration, theory, and application* (4th ed.). Wiley.

Ratts, M. J., Singh, A. A., Nassar-McMillan, S., Butler, S. K., & McCullough, J. R. (2016). Multicultural and social justice counseling competencies: Guidelines for the counseling profession. *Journal of Multicultural Counseling and Development, 44*(1), 28–48. https://doi.org/10.1002/jmcd.12035

Richeson, J. (2018, July/August). The paradox of diversity. *Association for Psychological Science Observer.* https://www.psychologicalscience.org/observer/the-paradox-of-diversity

Ridley, C. R., Mollen, D., Console, K., & Yin, C. (2021). Multicultural counseling competence: A construct in search of operationalization. *The Counseling Psychologist*, *49*(4), 504–533. https://doi.org/10.1177/0011000020988110

Ridley, C. R., Sahu, A., Console, K., Surya, S., Tran, V., Xie, S., & Yin, C. (2021). The process model of multicultural counseling competence. *The Counseling Psychologist*, *49*(4), 534–567. https://doi.org/10.1177/0011000021992339

Rodriguez, C. I., Cabaniss, D. L., Arbuckle, M. R., & Oquendo, M. A. (2008). The role of culture in psychodynamic psychotherapy: Parallel process resulting from cultural similarities between patient and therapist. *The American Journal of Psychiatry*, *165*(11), 1402–1406. https://doi.org/10.1176/appi.ajp.2008.08020215

Romo, R. (1986, Fall). George I. Sanchez and the civil rights movement: 1940–1960. *Berkeley La Raza Law Journal*, *1*(3), 342–362. https://doi.org/10.15779/Z385W8X

Roudinesco, E. (1990). *Jacques Lacan and Co.: A history of psychoanalysis in France, 1925–1985* (J. Mehlman, Trans.). Free Association Books.

Saguy, T., Dovidio, J. F., & Pratto, F. (2008). Beyond contact: Intergroup contact in the context of power relations. *Personality and Social Psychology Bulletin*, *34*(3), 432–445. https://doi.org/10.1177/0146167207311200

Sánchez, G. I. (1934). Bilingualism and mental measures. A word of caution. *Journal of Applied Psychology*, *18*(6), 765–772. https://doi.org/10.1037/h0072798

Schachter, A., Kimbro, R. T., & Gorman, B. K. (2012). Language proficiency and health status: Are bilingual immigrants healthier? *Journal of Health and Social Behavior*, *53*(1), 124–145. https://doi.org/10.1177/0022146511420570

Schneider, K. J., & Längle, A. (2012). The renewal of humanism in psychotherapy: Summary and conclusion. *Psychotherapy: Theory, Research, & Practice*, *49*(4), 480–481. https://doi.org/10.1037/a0028026

Searight, H. R., & Searight, B. K. (2009). Working with foreign language interpreters: Recommendations for psychological practice. *Professional Psychology: Research and Practice*, *40*(5), 444–451. https://doi.org/10.1037/a0016788

Sehgal, R., Saules, K., Young, A., Grey, M. J., Gillem, A. R., Nabors, N. A., Byrd, M. R., & Jefferson, S. (2011). Practicing what we know: Multicultural counseling competence among clinical psychology trainees and experienced multicultural psychologists. *Cultural Diversity & Ethnic Minority Psychology*, *17*(1), 1–10. https://doi.org/10.1037/a0021667

Seipel, A., & Sanders, S. (2016, March 22). *Cruz: "Empower law enforcement to patrol and secure Muslim neighborhoods."* NPR. https://www.npr.org/2016/03/22/471405546/u-s-officials-and-politicians-react-to-brussels-attacks

Shamsudheen, R. (2013). Out-group discrimination fuels anger, risk-taking and vigilance [Blog post]. *Brain Blogger.* http://www.brainblogger.com/2013/05/20/out-group-discrimination-fuels-anger-risk-taking-and-vigilance/

Sharf, J., Primavera, L. H., & Diener, M. J. (2010). Dropout and therapeutic alliance: A meta-analysis of adult individual psychotherapy. *Psychotherapy: Theory, Research, & Practice, 47*(4), 637–645. https://doi.org/10.1037/a0021175

Sharpless, B. A. (2018, December 22). *EPPP licensing exam discriminates against minorities.* https://www.modernpsychologist.com/eppp-licensing-exam-discriminates-against-minorities/

Sharpless, B. A. (2019). Are demographic variables associated with performance on the Examination for Professional Practice in Psychology (EPPP)? *The Journal of Psychology, 153*(2), 161–172. https://doi.org/10.1080/00223980.2018.1504739

Sharpless, B. A. (2021). Pass rates on the Examination for Professional Practice in Psychology (EPPP) according to demographic variables: A partial replication. *Training and Education in Professional Psychology, 15*(1), 18–22. https://doi.org/10.1037/tep0000301

Sheats, K. J., Irving, S. M., Mercy, J. A., Simon, T. R., Crosby, A. E., Ford, D. C., Merrick, M. T., Annor, F. B., & Morgan, R. E. (2018). Violence-related disparities experienced by Black youth and young adults: Opportunities for prevention. *American Journal of Preventive Medicine, 55*(4), 462–469. https://doi.org/10.1016/j.amepre.2018.05.017

Shen, Y.-J. (2016). A descriptive study of school counselors' play therapy experiences with the culturally diverse. *International Journal of Play Therapy, 25*(2), 54–63. https://doi.org/10.1037/pla0000017

Sherman, M. (2020, June 15). SCOTUS rules LGBTQ people protected from job discrimination. *PBS.* https://www.pbs.org/newshour/nation/scotus-rules-lgbt-people-protected-from-job-discrimination

Shin, R. Q., Smith, L. C., Welch, J. C., & Ezeofor, I. (2016). Is Allison more likely than Lakisha to receive a callback from counseling professionals? A racism audit study. *The Counseling Psychologist, 44*(8), 1187–1211. https://doi.org/10.1177/0011000016668814

Siegel, J. (2016). A *Journal of Family Social Work* conversation with Monica McGoldrick, LCSW. *Journal of Family Social Work, 19*(1), 56–64. https://doi.org/10.1080/10522158.2015.1133954

Silverstein, L. (2006). Integrating feminism and multiculturalism: Scientific fact or science fiction? *Professional Psychology: Research and Practice, 37*(1), 21–28. https://doi.org/10.1037/0735-7028.37.1.21

Smith, C., Denton, M. L., Faris, R., & Regnerus, M. (2002). Mapping American adolescent religious participation. *Journal for the Scientific Study of Religion, 41*(4), 597–612. https://doi.org/10.1111/1468-5906.00148

Smith, S. R., & Krishnamurthy, R. (Eds.). (2018). *Diversity-sensitive personality assessment.* Routledge. https://doi.org/10.4324/9780203551578

Smith, T. B., & Trimble, J. E. (2016). *Foundations of multicultural psychology: Research to inform effective practice*. American Psychological Association. https://doi.org/10.1037/14733-000

Snyder, C. R., Lopez, S. J., Shorey, H. S., Rand, K. L., & Feldman, D. B. (2003). Hope theory, measurements, and applications to school psychology. *School Psychology Quarterly, 18*(2), 122–139. https://doi.org/10.1521/scpq.18.2.122.21854

Soboroff, J. (2020). *Separated: An American tragedy*. HarperCollins.

State of Oregon, Board of Psychology. (n.d.). *Cultural competency continuing education*. https://www.oregon.gov/Psychology/Pages/CCCE.aspx

Steele, C. M. (1997). A threat in the air: How stereotypes shape intellectual identity and performance. *American Psychologist, 52*(6), 613–629. https://doi.org/10.1037/0003-066X.52.6.613

Steele, C. M. (2011). *Whistling Vivaldi: How stereotypes affect us and what we can do*. W. W. Norton.

Steele, C. M., & Aronson, J. (1995). Stereotype threat and the intellectual test performance of African Americans. *Journal of Personality and Social Psychology, 69*(5), 797–811. https://doi.org/10.1037/0022-3514.69.5.797

Steinhardt, M. A., Dubois, S. K., Brown, S. A., Harrison, L., Jr., Dolphin, K. E., Park, W., & Lehrer, H. M. (2015). Positivity and indicators of health among African Americans with diabetes. *American Journal of Health Behavior, 39*(1), 43–50. https://doi.org/10.5993/AJHB.39.1.5

Sternberg, R. J. (2014). The development of adaptive competence: Why cultural psychology is necessary and not just nice. *Developmental Review, 34*(3), 208–224. https://doi.org/10.1016/j.dr.2014.05.004

Substance Abuse and Mental Health Services Administration. (2015). *Racial/ethnic differences in mental health service use among adults* (HHS Publication No. SMA-15-4906). https://www.samhsa.gov/data/sites/default/files/MHServicesUseAmongAdults/MHServicesUseAmongAdults.pdf

Sue, D. W. (2003). *Overcoming our racism: The journey to liberation*. Jossey-Bass. https://doi.org/10.1002/9780787979690

Sue, D. W., Alsaidi, S., Awad, M. N., Glaeser, E., Calle, C. Z., & Mendez, N. (2019). Disarming racial microaggressions: Microintervention strategies for targets, White allies, and bystanders. *American Psychologist, 74*(1), 128–142. https://doi.org/10.1037/amp0000296

Sue, D. W., Arredondo, P., & McDavis, R. J. (1992). Multicultural counseling competencies and standards: A call to the profession. *Journal of Counseling and Development, 70*(4), 477–486. https://doi.org/10.1002/j.1556-6676.1992.tb01642.x

Sue, D. W., Ivey, A., & Pedersen, P. (2007). *Theory of multicultural counseling & therapy*. Cengage Learning Press.

Sue, D. W., & Sue, D. (2003). *Counseling the culturally diverse: Theory and practice* (4th ed.). Wiley.

Sue, D. W., & Sue, D. (2008). *Counseling the culturally diverse: Theory and practice* (5th ed.). Wiley.

Sue, D. W., & Sue, D. (2013). *Counseling the culturally diverse: Theory and practice* (6th ed.). Wiley.

Sue, D. W., & Sue, D. (2016). *Counseling the culturally diverse: Theory and practice* (7th ed.). Wiley.

Sue, D. W., & Sue, D. (2019). *Counseling the culturally diverse: Theory and practice* (8th ed.). Wiley.

Sue, S. (1998). In search of cultural competence in psychotherapy and counseling. *American Psychologist, 53*(4), 440–448. https://doi.org/10.1037/0003-066X.53.4.440

Sue, S. (1999). Science, ethnicity, and bias: Where have we gone wrong? *American Psychologist, 54*(12), 1070–1077. https://doi.org/10.1037/0003-066X.54.12.1070

Sue, S. (2006). Cultural competency: From philosophy to research and practice. *Journal of Community Psychology, 34*(2), 237–245. https://doi.org/10.1002/jcop.20095

Sue, S. (2009). Ethnic minority psychology: Struggles and triumphs. *Cultural Diversity & Ethnic Minority Psychology, 15*(4), 409–415. https://doi.org/10.1037/a0017559

Sue, S., Zane, N., Nagayama Hall, G. C., & Berger, L. K. (2009). The case for cultural competency in psychotherapeutic interventions. *Annual Review of Psychology, 60*(1), 525–548. https://doi.org/10.1146/annurev.psych.60.110707.163651

Sufrin, J. (2019, November 5). 3 things to know: Cultural humility [Blog post]. *Hogg Blog.* https://hogg.utexas.edu/3-things-to-know-cultural-humility

Summers, F. (2014). Ethnic invisibility, identity, and the analytic process. *Psychoanalytic Psychology, 31*(3), 410–425. https://doi.org/10.1037/a0037330

Swenson, C. (1998). Clinical social work's contribution to a social justice perspective. *Social Work, 43*(6), 527–537. https://doi.org/10.1093/sw/43.6.527

Swift, J. K., Callahan, J. L., Tompkins, K. A., Connor, D. R., & Dunn, R. (2015). A delay-discounting measure of preference for racial/ethnic matching in psychotherapy. *Psychotherapy, 52*(3), 315–320. https://doi.org/10.1037/pst0000019

Swift, J. K., & Greenberg, R. P. (2014). A treatment by disorder meta-analysis of dropout from psychotherapy. *Journal of Psychotherapy Integration, 24*(3), 193–207. https://doi.org/10.1037/a0037512

Tao, K. W., Owen, J., Pace, B. T., & Imel, Z. E. (2015). A meta-analysis of multicultural competencies and psychotherapy process and outcome. *Journal of Counseling Psychology, 62*(3), 337–350. https://doi.org/10.1037/cou0000086

Tate, K., Torres Rivera, E., Brown, E., & Skaitis, L. (2013). Foundations for liberation: Social justice, liberation psychology and counseling. *The Journal of Psychology*, *47*(3), 373–382.

Taylor, C., Clifford, A., & Franklin, A. (2013). Color preferences are not universal. *Journal of Experimental Psychology: General*, *142*(4), 1015–1027. https://doi.org/10.1037/a0030273

Taylor, K.-Y. (2019). *Race for profit: How banks and the real estate industry undermined Black homeownership*. University of North Carolina Press.

Taylor, K.-Y. (2020, June 8). How do we change America? *The New Yorker*. https://www.newyorker.com/news/our-columnists/how-do-we-change-america

Taylor, R. J., Chatters, L. M., Jayakody, R., & Levin, J. S. (1996). Black and White differences in religious participation: A multi-sample comparison. *Journal for the Scientific Study of Religion*, *35*(4), 403–410. https://doi.org/10.2307/1386415

Taylor, S. (2015, September 25). Transpersonal psychology: Exploring the farther reaches of human nature [Blog post]. *Psychology Today*. https://www.psychologytoday.com/us/blog/out-the-darkness/201509/transpersonal-psychology

Tervalon, M., & Murray-García, J. (1998). Cultural humility versus cultural competence: A critical distinction in defining physician training outcomes in multicultural education. *Journal of Health Care for the Poor and Underserved*, *9*(2), 117–125. https://doi.org/10.1353/hpu.2010.0233

Theorell, T. (2020). COVID-19 and working conditions in health care. *Psychotherapy and Psychosomatics*, *89*(4), 193–194. https://doi.org/10.1159/000507765

Thrift, E., & Sugarman, J. (2019). What is social justice? Implications for psychology. *Journal of Theoretical and Philosophical Psychology*, *39*(1), 1–17. https://doi.org/10.1037/teo0000097

Tillich, P. (1957). *Systematic theology: Existence and the Christ* (Vol. 2). University of Chicago Press.

Title VII of the Civil Rights Act of 1964. https://www.eeoc.gov/statutes/title-vii-civil-rights-act-1964

Tolin, D. F., McKay, D., Forman, E. M., Klonsky, D. E., & Thombs, D. E. (2015). Empirically supported treatment: Recommendations for a new model. *Clinical Psychology: Science and Practice*, *22*(4), 317–338. https://doi.org/10.1111/cpsp.12122

Tori, C. D., & Bilmes, M. (2002). Multiculturalism and psychoanalytic psychology: The validation of a defense mechanisms measure in an Asian population. *Psychoanalytic Psychology*, *19*(4), 701–721. https://doi.org/10.1037/0736-9735.19.4.701

Trimble, J. E., & Clearing-Sky, M. (2009). An historical profile of American Indians and Alaska Natives in psychology. *Cultural Diversity & Ethnic Minority Psychology*, *15*(4), 338–351. https://doi.org/10.1037/a0015112

Tseng, W. S., & Streltzer, J. (Eds.). (2004). *Cultural competence in clinical psychiatry.* American Psychiatric Publishing.

Tummala-Narra, P. (2009). The relevance of a psychoanalytic perspective in exploring religious and spiritual identity in psychotherapy. *Psychoanalytic Psychology, 26*(1), 83–95. https://doi.org/10.1037/a0014673

Tummala-Narra, P. (2016). *Psychoanalytic theory and cultural competence in psychotherapy.* American Psychological Association. https://doi.org/10.1037/14800-000

Tylor, E. B. (1920). *Primitive culture: Researches into the development of mythology, philosophy, religion, art, and custom* (6th ed., Vol. 1). Murray.

U.S. Census Bureau. (2015). *American community survey.* https://www.census.gov/acs/www/data/data-tables-and-tools/data-profiles/2015

U.S. Census Bureau. (2017). *Facts-for-features: Hispanic heritage month.* https://www.census.gov/newsroom/facts-for-features/2017/hispanic-heritage.html

U.S. Census Bureau, Public Information Office. (2012, December 12). *U.S. Census Bureau projections show a slower growing, older, more diverse nation a half century from now* [Press release]. https://www.census.gov/newsroom/releases/archives/population/cb12-243.html

U.S. Department of Health and Human Services. (2001). *Mental health: Culture, race and ethnicity—A supplement to Mental health: A report of the Surgeon General.* https://www.ncbi.nlm.nih.gov/books/NBK44243/

U.S. Department of Health and Human Services Office of Minority Health. (2021a). *Mental and behavioral health—African Americans.* https://minorityhealth.hhs.gov/omh/browse.aspx?lvl=4&lvlid=24

U.S. Department of Health and Human Services Office of Minority Health. (2021b). *Mental and behavioral health—American Indians/Alaska Natives.* https://www.minorityhealth.hhs.gov/omh/browse.aspx?lvl=4&lvlid=39

U.S. Department of Health and Human Services Office of Minority Health. (2021c). *Mental and behavioral health—Asian Americans.* https://minorityhealth.hhs.gov/omh/browse.aspx?lvl=4&lvlid=54

U.S. Department of Health and Human Services Office of Minority Health. (2021d). *Mental and behavioral health—Hispanics.* https://minorityhealth.hhs.gov/omh/browse.aspx?lvl=4&lvlid=69

U.S. Department of Justice, Federal Bureau of Investigation, Uniform Crime Reporting Program. (2016). *2016 hate crime statistics.* https://ucr.fbi.gov/hate-crime/2016/topic-pages/incidentsandoffenses

Van Den Bergh, N. (2004). Getting a piece of the pie: Cultural competence for GLBT employees at the workplace. *Journal of Human Behavior in the Social Environment, 8*(2–3), 55–73. https://doi.org/10.1300/J137v08n02_04

Vasquez, M. J. T. (2007a). Cultural difference and the therapeutic alliance: An evidence-based analysis. *American Psychologist, 62*(8), 878–885. https://doi.org/10.1037/0003-066X.62.8.878

Vasquez, M. J. T. (2007b). Ethics for a diverse world. In J. Frew & M. D. Spiegler (Eds.), *Contemporary psychotherapies for a diverse world* (pp. 20–40). Houghton Mifflin/Lahaska Press.

Vasquez, M. J. T. (2012). Psychology and social justice: Why we do what we do. *American Psychologist, 67*(5), 337–346. https://doi.org/10.1037/a0029232

Vasquez, M. J. T., & de las Fuentes, C. (1999). American-born Asian, African, Latina, and American Indian adolescent girls: Challenges and strengths. In N. G. Johnson, M. C. Roberts, & J. Worell (Eds.), *Beyond appearance: A new look at adolescent girls* (pp. 151–173). American Psychological Association. https://doi.org/10.1037/10325-006

Vasquez, M. J. T., & Heppner, P. P. (2017). Counseling psychologists. In R. J. Sternberg (Ed.), *Career paths in psychology: Where your degree can take you* (pp. 189–210). American Psychological Association. https://doi.org/10.1037/15960-013

Vazquez, L. A. (2014). Integration of multicultural and psychoanalytic concepts: A review of three case examples with Women of Color. *Psychoanalytic Psychology, 31*(3), 435–448. https://doi.org/10.1037/a0036341

Vontress, C. E. (2008). Foreword. In P. B. Pedersen, J. G. Draguns, W. J. Lonner, & J. E. Trimble (Eds.), *Counseling across cultures* (6th ed.). Sage.

Wakefield, J. C. (1988a). Psychotherapy, distributive justice, and social work: Part 1. Distributive justice as a conceptual framework for social work. *The Social Service Review, 62*(2), 187–210. https://doi.org/10.1086/644542

Wakefield, J. C. (1988b). Psychotherapy, distributive justice, and social work: Part 2. Psychotherapy and the pursuit of justice. *The Social Service Review, 62*(3), 353–382. https://doi.org/10.1086/644555

Walker, M. (2020). *When getting along is not enough: Reconstructing race in our lives and relationships.* Teachers College Press/Columbia University.

Walsh, R., & Vaughan, F. (1993). On transpersonal definitions. *Journal of Transpersonal Psychology, 25*(2), 199–207.

Wampold, B. E. (2000). Outcomes of individual counseling and psychotherapy: Empirical evidence addressing two fundamental questions. In S. D. Brown & R. W. Lent (Eds.), *Handbook of counseling psychology* (3rd ed., pp. 571–600). Wiley.

Wampold, B. E. (2015). How important are the common factors in psychotherapy? An update. *World Psychiatry, 14*(3), 270–277. https://doi.org/10.1002/wps.20238

Wampold, B. E., & Imel, Z. E. (2015). *The great psychotherapy debate: The evidence for what makes psychotherapy work* (2nd ed.). Routledge. https://doi.org/10.4324/9780203582015

Wang, Q. (2008). Emotion knowledge and autobiographical memory across the preschool years: A cross-cultural longitudinal investigation. *Cognition, 108*(1), 117–135. https://doi.org/10.1016/j.cognition.2008.02.002

Wang, Q. (2016). Why should we all be cultural psychologists? Lessons from the study of social cognition. *Perspectives on Psychological Science, 11*(5), 583–596. https://doi.org/10.1177/1745691616645552

Welland, C., & Ribner, N. (2007). *Healing from violence: Latino men's journey to a new masculinity.* Springer Publishing Co.

Weng, H. Y., Fox, A. S., Shackman, A. J., Stodola, D. E., Caldwell, J. Z. K., Olson, M. C., Rogers, G. M., & Davidson, R. J. (2013). Compassion training alters altruism and neural responses to suffering. *Psychological Science, 24*(7), 1171–1180. https://doi.org/10.1177/0956797612469537

Whaley, A. L., & Davis, K. E. (2007). Cultural competence and evidence-based practice in mental health services: A complementary perspective. *American Psychologist, 62*(6), 563–574. https://doi.org/10.1037/0003-066X.62.6.563

White, C. (2007, February 12). Horace Mann Bond (1904–1972). *Blackpast.org.* https://www.blackpast.org/african-american-history/bond-horace-mann-1904-1972/

Williams, M., Powers, M., Yun, Y. G., & Foa, E. (2010). Minority participation in randomized controlled trials for obsessive-compulsive disorder. *Journal of Anxiety Disorders, 24*(2), 171–177. https://doi.org/10.1016/j.janxdis.2009.11.004

Winkeljohn Black, S., Drinane, J. M., Owen, J., DeBlaere, C., & Davis, D. (2021). Integrating spirituality as a multicultural component into time-limited psychotherapy: Two case studies. *Professional Psychology: Research and Practice, 52*(2), 121–129. https://doi.org/10.1037/pro0000369

Wintersteen, M., Mensinger, J., & Diamond, G. (2005). Do gender and racial differences between patient and therapist affect therapeutic alliance and treatment retention in adolescents? *Professional Psychology: Research and Practice, 36*(4), 400–408. https://doi.org/10.1037/0735-7028.36.4.400

Withers, B. (1972). Use me [Song]. *Lyrics.com.* https://www.lyrics.com/lyric/154718/Bill+Withers

Wolsko, C., Park, B., & Judd, C. M. (2006). Considering the tower of Babel: Correlates of assimilation and multiculturalism among ethnic minority and majority groups in the United States. *Social Justice Research, 19*(3), 277–306. https://doi.org/10.1007/s11211-006-0014-8

Wong, Y. J., Wang, S.-Y., & Klann, E. M. (2018). The emperor with no clothes: A critique of collectivism and individualism. *Archives of Scientific Psychology*, 6(1), 251–260. https://doi.org/10.1037/arc0000059

World Health Organization. (1993). *The ICD-10 classification of mental and behavioural disorders*. https://icd.who.int/

Wu, C. H., Erickson, S. R., Piette, J. D., & Balkrishnan, R. (2012). Mental health resource utilization and health care costs associated with race and comorbid anxiety among Medicaid enrollees with major depressive disorder. *Journal of the National Medical Association*, 104(1–2), 78–88. https://doi.org/10.1016/S0027-9684(15)30121-8

Xiao, H., Castonguay, L. G., Janis, R. A., Youn, S. J., Hayes, J. A., & Locke, B. D. (2017). Therapist effects on dropout from a college counseling center practice research network. *Journal of Counseling Psychology*, 64(4), 424–431. https://doi.org/10.1037/cou0000208

Yakushko, O. (2010). Clinical work with limited English proficiency clients: A phenomenological exploration. *Professional Psychology: Research and Practice*, 41(5), 449–455. https://doi.org/10.1037/a0020996

Yeager, K. A., & Bauer-Wu, S. (2013). Cultural humility: Essential foundation for clinical researchers. *Applied Nursing Research*, 26(4), 251–256. https://doi.org/10.1016/j.apnr.2013.06.008

Yee, T., Ceballos, P., & Swan, A. (2019). Examining the trends of play therapy articles: A 10-year content analysis. *International Journal of Play Therapy*, 28(4), 250–260. https://doi.org/10.1037/pla0000103

Zaker, B. S., & Boostanipoor, A. (2016). Multiculturalism in counseling and therapy: Marriage and family issues. *International Journal of Psychology and Counselling*, 8(5), 53–57. https://doi.org/10.5897/IJPC2016.0388

Zhang, W. R., Wang, K., Yin, L., Zhao, W. F., Xue, Q., Peng, M., Min, B. Q., Tian, Q., Leng, H. X., Du, J. L., Chang, H., Yang, Y., Li, W., Shangguan, F. F., Yan, T. Y., Dong, H. Q., Han, Y., Wang, Y. P., Cosci, F., & Wang, H. X. (2020). Mental health and psychosocial problems of medical health workers during the COVID-19 epidemic in China. *Psychotherapy and Psychosomatics*, 89(4), 242–250. https://doi.org/10.1159/000507639

Index

About the Authors

Melba J. T. Vasquez, PhD, is in independent practice in Austin, Texas. One of the most exciting periods in her career was when she served as president of the American Psychological Association (APA) in 2011. She is the first Latina and Woman of Color to serve in that role of 120 APA presidencies. Her theme for the 2011 APA convention was social justice. Her special presidential initiatives included examination of psychology's contributions to the challenges in society, including immigration, discrimination, and educational disparities.

Dr. Vasquez also served a term on the APA Board of Directors. She is a former president of the Texas Psychological Association and of APA Divisions 35 (Society for the Psychology of Women) and 17 (Society of Counseling Psychology). She is a cofounder of APA Division 45 (Society for the Psychological Study of Culture, Ethnicity and Race), and of the National Multicultural Conference and Summit. She is a fellow of 11 divisions of the APA and holds the Diplomate of the American Board of Professional Psychology.

Dr. Vasquez obtained her doctorate in counseling psychology from the University of Texas at Austin in 1978. Before becoming a psychologist, she taught middle school. She has served as parliamentarian for the 2021 APA President Jennifer Kelly and for the 2020 APA President Sandra Shullman. Dr. Vasquez served a term on the APA Needs, Assessment, Slating and Campaigns Committee (NASCC), and several terms on the Board of Trustees of the American Psychological Foundation.

She is a coauthor of six editions of *Ethics in Psychotherapy and Counseling: A Practical Guide*, of *How to Survive and Thrive as a Therapist: Information, Ideas, and Resources for Psychologists in Practice*, and of the *APA Ethics Code Commentary and Case Illustrations*. Dr. Vasquez has also published about 100 book chapters and journal articles in the areas of professional ethics, ethnic minority psychology, psychology of women, counseling and psychotherapy, and leadership. She has served on numerous editorial boards.

Dr. Vasquez has been honored with more than 50 awards for distinguished professional contributions, career service, leadership, advocacy, and mentorship.

She is married to Jim H. Miller, a big supporter of her career. She very much values the full support of her friends and extended family, including her stepdaughter and six siblings and their families. She is grateful that despite having only elementary educations, both her parents were politically involved at the grassroots level, engaged in civil rights activities, and articulated a strong belief in and support for education. She appreciates that they guided her into productive social justice advocacy all her life.

Josephine D. Johnson, PhD, has a private practice in Farmington Hills, Michigan, providing services to adolescents, adults, and families, and clinical supervision to doctoral and master's level psychologists. She has been a long-time consultant to community mental health agencies, served many years as a specialist to residential treatment facilities, and has been a consultant to businesses, schools, churches, and to a university counseling and psychological services program. Dr. Johnson received a BA in psychology from Northwestern University, and a master's in school psychology and doctorate in clinical psychology from the University of Detroit. She is a trustee for the American Insurance Trust and has been an officer on the board of the Metro Detroit Association of Black Psychologists. Dr. Johnson served as president of the Michigan Psychological Association and received its "Psychologist of the Year" award in 2009; she also received their Beth Clark Service Award in 2018 and served for 14 years as Michigan's Federal Advocacy Coordinator.

Dr. Johnson served on the American Psychological Association's (APA's) Board of Directors, Committee for the Advancement of Professional Practice, and several other boards and committees. She chaired the APA Task Force on the Implementation of the Multicultural Guidelines and was a member of the Task Force on Evidence-Based Practice in Psychology. Dr. Johnson was awarded an APA Presidential Citation (2021) by APA President Jennifer Kelly, the APA State Leadership Award (2017), the Psychologists in Independent Practice Public Service Award (2016), and the APA Committee of State Leaders Diversity Delegates Recognition Award (2013). She is a graduate of the Chamber of Commerce's Leadership Detroit program. She has conducted numerous workshops and trainings on multiculturalism, including a cultural sensitivity retreat experience for high school girls for 20 years. For more information, visit her website (JohnsonBehavioralHealth.com).

About the Series Editor

Matt Englar-Carlson, PhD, is a professor of counseling and director of the Center for Boys and Men at California State University–Fullerton. A Fellow of the American Psychological Association (APA), Dr. Englar-Carlson's scholarship focuses on training helping professionals to work more effectively with boys and men across the full range of human diversity. His publications and presentations are focused on men and masculinities, social justice and diversity issues in psychological training and practice, and theories of psychotherapy. Dr. Englar-Carlson coedited the books *In the Room With Men: A Casebook of Therapeutic Change, Counseling Troubled Boys: A Guidebook for Professionals, Beyond the 50-Minute Hour: Therapists Involved in Meaningful Social Action,* and *A Counselor's Guide to Working With Men,* and he was featured in the APA-produced video *Engaging Men in Psychotherapy.* He was named Researcher of the Year, Professional of the Year, and he received the Professional Service award from the Society for the Psychological Study of Men and Masculinities, and was one of the core authors of the *APA Guidelines for Professional Psychological Practice With Boys and Men.* As a clinician, Dr. Englar-Carlson has worked with children, adults, and families in school, community, and university mental health settings. He is the coauthor of *Adlerian Psychotherapy,* which is part of the Theories of Psychotherapy Series.